LEADING with MASTERY and HEART

The Coaching Companion for Thriving Nurse Leaders

LEADING with MASTERY and HEART

The Coaching Companion for Thriving Nurse Leaders

CATHERINE ROBINSON-WALKER, MBA

Master Certified Coach
President, The Leadership Studio®
Walnut Creek, CA
www.leadershipstudio.com

ELSEVIER

Elsevier
3251 Riverport Lane
St. Louis, Missouri 63043

Notices

Library of Congress Control Number: 2019952830

Executive Content Strategist: Yvonne Alexopoulos
Content Development Specialist: Brooke Kannady
Publishing Services Manager: Shereen Jameel
Senior Project Manager: Umarani Natarajan
Design Direction: Bridget Hoette

Printed in the United States of America

Last digit is the print number: 9   8   7   6   5   4   3   2   1

Working together
to grow libraries in
developing countries

www.elsevier.com • www.bookaid.org

To all nurses, for your service and dedication to humanity's well-being.

Catherine Robinson-Walker, MBA, MCC, has thoroughly enjoyed working with nurses throughout her career. Her lifelong professional focus has been in the fields of leadership development and executive coaching in health care. Cathy has 25 years of executive leadership experience in complex health organizations, national associations, commissions, and academic institutions. She has served nurse leaders, physicians, chief executives, management teams, and other senior healthcare staff as a Master Certified executive coach, strategic consultant, team facilitator, keynote and workshop speaker, and author.

Since the 1980s, a central focal point of Cathy's work has been providing professional and personal development tools and support for nurse leaders. This work has given her a rich understanding of the opportunities and challenges that nurse managers and leaders face every day. Over the years, Cathy has been invited to direct and co-create numerous leadership programs for nurses, including most notably the initial funding effort to create **The Florence Nightingale Museum of Nursing in London, England.** Cathy spearheaded the 10-day leadership program that launched the Florence Nightingale Museum's building campaign in 1986.

She has also headed other distinguished nursing leadership programs, including:

- **The Network Institute for Patient Care Executives** (aka The Western Network Institute for Nursing Executives), a week-long program held at the University of California Berkeley.
- **The Center for Nursing Leadership Program**, a year-long program developed in collaboration with the American Organization for Nursing Leadership (then called the American Organization of Nurse Executives).
- **The Executive Coaching Resource Center**, an online coaching resource center for members of the American Organization for Nursing Leadership.
- **The Executive Coaching Service**, sponsored and funded by the National Council of State Boards of Nursing in the United States.

Cathy's first book, *Women and Leadership in Health Care: The Journey to Authenticity and Power*, was a Jossey-Bass health series best seller. Her second book, *Leading Valiantly in Healthcare*, published by Sigma Theta Tau, also received wide acclaim. In addition, Cathy is the author of numerous continuing education courses and articles. She has also been the author of *The Coaching Forum*, a featured column devoted to the challenges of nursing leadership in *Nurse Leader*, the official journal of the American Organization for Nursing Leadership/the American Hospital Association.

For 18 years, Cathy was the founding CEO of the Network for Healthcare Management, a multinational fifteen-university consortium of graduate programs in health management. These included the University of California Berkeley, the Kellogg School at Northwestern University, and the Wharton School at the University of Pennsylvania. In addition, she held Executive Director roles with the Chicago-based Joint Commission, the Public Health Institute and the California Health Collaborative.

Cathy first earned the designation of Master Certified Coach, the International Coach Federation's highest level of achievement, in 2005. She has served as a member of the Leadership Team for the Hudson Institute of Coaching since 2001, and she has also served as one of a small cadre of executive coaches for the National Center for Healthcare Leadership.

Cathy has earned a number of other certifications for competencies that she employs in her work, including those related to the Enneagram and emotional intelligence. She has worked in multiple capacities with leaders and teams from a variety of healthcare organizations, such as the American Nurses Association, Children's Hospital of Orange County (CHOC), the National Council of State Boards of Nursing, the American Organization for Nursing Leadership, The Association of California Nurse Leaders, the National Cancer Institute, Sutter Health and many others.

Cathy has received considerable recognition throughout her career, including being named "Woman of the Year" by Women Healthcare Executives of Northern California/American College of Healthcare Executives, "Friend of Nursing" by the Association of California Nurse Leaders and "Honorary Member" by Sigma Theta Tau, the international honor society for nurses.

Cathy lives in the San Francisco Bay Area with her husband and their two cats, Casey and Jet.

Catherine Robinson-Walker, MBA, MCC
President, The Leadership Studio®
www.leadershipstudio.com
cathy@leadershipstudio.com
925-946-1582

FOREWORD

A formulaic approach to one's professional development will not be successful in today's complex and rapidly evolving healthcare environment. Leadership today requires deep reflection, authenticity, and a balance between courage and humility. Cathy Robinson-Walker has always generously helped nurses understand leadership as an art as well as a science and infuses this book with guidance on leading both with mastery *and* heart. She well understands that thriving as a leader involves tapping into deep expertise and humanity, fully utilizing one's intellect and energy. This applies to the novice as well as the seasoned leader—all can learn and benefit from self-reflection.

This book does not have to be read cover to cover, in sequential order, or even by sections. It can be picked up and read randomly or by focusing on topics of interest. When things are going well, it will remind you to tap into your expertise and courage to fully express the depth of your leadership. At those desolate moments of vulnerability when you as a leader are uncertain about what direction to head and how to best proceed, this book will provide guidance and insights about a path forward. In all moments, it will encourage you to examine where you hide your courage and stimulate your thinking about leadership. It will help you confront those who want to lead by domination and to co-create magnificent outcomes with those who want to collaborate. We do not lead in isolation; we should not learn in isolation either. Any way you approach reading the material, the content will give you something to think about, inspire you, and bring out the best of yourself as a leader.

The book focuses on the essence of our practice as nurse leaders and is based on years of Cathy's work as a senior executive and her work coaching top-level nurse executive leaders. The best leaders are open to ongoing coaching and learning. Coaches provide a safe space for honesty and exploration, asking compassionate and brutally honest questions to support a reflective practice. As a result, the material in this book provides a resource to internalize the practices of coaching to direct your own reflection. You are never done with your development. Looking at your practice from multiple perspectives lets you build depth and resilience.

Your actions as a leader carry wide and far. You never know when or how your leadership moments will have an impact. Small, seemingly insignificant interactions and observations may create lasting impressions on a colleague about which you will hear years later. Our actions as leaders are never insignificant. Reflections in our practice helps us see potential and patterns and constantly build our personal leadership persona.

The generous reflections and lessons shared by Cathy will support you to be a leader who serves with mastery and heart and to wisely use your power to create a long-lasting impact on the world. As Cathy describes, as a leader you have a huge wake with ripples that continue long after you have gone.

Pamela Thompson, RN, MS, FAAN
American Organization for Nursing Leadership CEO Emeritus

Marla J. Weston, PhD, RN, FAAN
American Nurses Association Enterprise CEO Emeritus

INTRODUCTION

As a nurse, you are the lifeblood of health care delivery. You are also its heart. This is true throughout the world, and in delivery systems of every kind. Certainly, you join with important others from different disciplines, and yes, you collaborate with those individuals to optimally serve patients and their families. But it is you, the nurse, who administers and oversees the care of patients on a day in and day out basis. It is you, the nurse, who understands that providing high-quality care every day requires extensive knowledge, skill, and dedication. It is you whose work fulfills a critical human and social need for care, attention, and well-being.

As a nurse who leads, or aspires to lead, you direct, influence, and make decisions that profoundly affect people's lives—patients, their families, other caregivers, managers, and staff. As a nurse who incorporates management and leadership into your work, you impact the very systems in which people receive their care. Your role requires that you face exceptional complexity on a daily basis. It requires extraordinary focus, steadfastness, and compassion as you balance the many—sometimes competing—priorities that emerge every day. It requires that you lead with mastery and heart.

Leading with Mastery and Heart: The Coaching Companion for Thriving Nurse Leaders is intended to be a "just-in-time" offering to support you as you address the unique demands of nurse leadership. I assembled the articles in this collection at the request of readers of *The Coaching Forum*, the featured column that appeared in *Nurse Leader*, the official magazine for the American Organization for Nursing Leadership (AONL),[a] for many years.[b] Whether you are early in your nursing career, you are a manager, or you are a thriving nurse leader right now, I hope you will consult this leadership resource often to gain new perspectives and fresh approaches to the leadership challenges that arise in your life.

WHAT DOES "MASTERY" MEAN FOR A NURSE LEADER?

Mastery is neither a lofty ideal nor a static state. Mastery is not a single destination, a place we reach through position or age. Rather, true mastery is about continual practice of our chosen craft and perpetual refinement of our talents. By definition, a master's skills are frequently stretched and repeatedly challenged. A true master's experience evolves and deepens in every circumstance.

~ From **The Coaching Forum** *column in the first issue of* **Nurse Leader**[c]

Mastery is a continuous journey toward excellence, one that can be undertaken by nurses at any stage of their nursing and leadership career. The AONL states that "to master the art and science of being a nurse leader is to master the competencies and skills involved in nurse leadership."[d] Thus, mastery also means competence, including a common set of nurse executive competencies captured in a model developed in 2004 by the Healthcare Leadership Alliance.[e] *Leading with Mastery and Heart* speaks to many of these competencies, including communication and relationship building, influencing, personal journey disciplines, succession planning, change management, accountability, and career management and planning.[f]

---

[a]Formerly known as The American Organization of Nurse Executives (AONE)
[b]From 2006 through 2018.

---

[c]*Nurse Leader*, April 2006.
[d]Per the AONL website, "Nurse Leaders in Executive Practice," 2015, citing the work they did in 2004.
[e]"The AONE Nurse Executive Competencies detail the skills knowledge and abilities that guide the practice of nurse leaders in executive practice regardless of their educational level, title or setting. The competencies are captured in a model developed in 2004 by the Healthcare Leadership Alliance that identify the common core set of competency domains for health care leadership: communication and relationship management; knowledge of the health care environment; leadership; professionalism; business skills and principles." Per the AONL website, "Nurse Leaders in Executive Practice," 2015.
[f]As above, from the Nurse Leaders in Executive Practice competencies noted on the website per the previous footnote.

WHAT DOES "HEART" MEAN FOR A NURSE LEADER?

The root of the word "heart" or "heorte" means soul, spirit, will, courage, and even the mind, in Old English.[g] In the symbolic world, "heart" is often used to mean the moral, emotional, spiritual, and even intellectual substance of a person.

Cultural anthropologist Dr. Angeles Arrien, whose wisdom inspired one of my columns in *Nurse Leader*,[h] elegantly embraces the heart within Healer as one of the four essential energies. In her book *The Four Fold Way*,[i] she wrote:

> *The archetype of the Healer is a universal mythic structure that all human beings experience. Among indigenous cultures the Healer supports the principle of paying attention to what has heart and meaning. Healers in all major traditions recognize that the power of love is the most potent healing force available to all human beings. Effective Healers from any culture are those who extend the arms of love: acknowledgement, acceptance, recognition, validation, and gratitude.*

Dr. Arrien also stated that, "etymologically, the word heart means 'the ability to stand by one's heart or to stand by one's core.' Whenever we exhibit courage, we demonstrate the healing power of paying attention to what has heart and meaning."

True healers lead with heart—with courage, recognition, validation, and gratitude. As much as mastery, these practices are essential to the success of the nurse leader.

LEADING WITH MASTERY AND HEART EVERY DAY

My years of coaching experience with nurses and nurse leaders assure me of two fundamental truths: no matter where you are in your nursing career, you already possess the potential to lead masterfully; you also have the capacity to lead with heart.

Leading with mastery and heart means that you are pursuing excellence in the science and art of leadership while staying in touch with and connected to what has heart and meaning for you. This is a fulfilling yet challenging journey for nurse leaders and managers who face a multitude of specific yet universal leadership demands every day. Nurse leaders are tasked with strategic and operational responsibilities that can stress their abilities to be thoughtful, reflective, and insightful in their approaches to their work. Many times, nurse leaders are—correctly—caught up in the significant obligations of their positions rather than stepping back and allowing themselves time to think through the best approaches to their priorities.

In offering this collection, it is my purpose to give you, the nurse leader, immediate access to practical, proven strategies for the complexities you face. The stories in this collection are dedicated to your learning, your mastery, and your ability to focus on what has heart and meaning for you. Most of these stories are "tales from the front." That is, they were inspired by nurses, nurse managers, and leaders just like you. Although identities are intermingled and disguised, each narrative is based on these leaders' real professional and personal circumstances. Each is informed by the ways in which they faced sometimes significant discord, yet still found the means to move forward and succeed. Through their experiences, I hope you will gain new perspective on what's working and not working in your own leadership life, and find fresh solutions and practices that support you in becoming the thriving leader you are meant to be.

HOW TO FIND WHAT YOU NEED

This collection is organized into five sections, each building on the one that precedes it. You can pick it up anywhere, turning to the section or article that is most relevant to you in the moment, or you can start from the beginning.

The first section, Knowing Who You Are as a Leader, is dedicated to the important work of self-awareness and self-management, and it includes four parts: Introspection and Learning; True North: Your Values; Emotional Triggers and Ghosts; and Compassion and Care for Yourself.

The second section, Building Relationships That Thrive, focuses on what it takes to create and sustain strong and mutually beneficial professional partnerships. Its three parts are: Influence, Communication, and Respect; Relationship Landmines and Let-Downs; and Loving Your Team—No Matter What.

The third section is about Leading Change, an essential skill for leaders at all levels. Its three parts are Ready or Not, Change Is Here; Change Happens—So Does Resistance; and When the Change Maker Is You.

---

[g]www.etymonline.com.

[h]Please see the Appendix for the complete article dedicated to the wisdom of Dr. Angeles Arrien.

[i]*The Four Fold Way: Walking the Paths of Warrior, Teacher, Healer and Visionary*. HarperOne, 1993.

The fourth section, Claiming Your Power and Your Place, is dedicated to increasing your power and influence as a masterful leader. It contains two parts: It's Your Turn to Lead and Navigating Power Detractors.

Finally, the fifth section, Leading with Mastery and Heart, builds on the sections that preceded it, and it concentrates on leveraging your impact and legacy. It has two parts: Developing Others and Being a Role Model.

MY WISH FOR YOU

As a nurse who leads, you and your peers have served as inspiration for me throughout my health care career. It is my hope that I can return that inspiration many-fold in this collection of your stories, your challenges, and your successes. May you lead masterfully, always remembering to focus on what has heart and meaning for you.

ACKNOWLEDGMENTS

You would not be reading *Leading with Mastery and Heart* were it not for the countless nurse leaders who have worked with me throughout my career. The spirit and the lessons in this collection would be far less compelling were it not for their honesty, their vulnerability, and their willingness to dig deep to find and maintain their, courage, focus, and grit. I am not just indebted to them for the gift of our journeys together; I am indebted to them for inspiration to make ever stronger my commitment to provide them with solace, safety, and partnership as they pursued leadership mastery on their own terms.

Being invited to create a column called *The Coaching Forum* was a delightful surprise offered to me in 2006 by the founding editor of *Nurse Leader*, Dr. Roxane Spitzer. With her blessing and with the support of my *Nurse Leader* editorial board colleagues, along with Roxane's successor, Dr. Rose Sherman, I was given a venue to share best practices, intractable challenges, and—despite it all—the successful ways forward that nurse leaders were creating through the years. Although their stories are combined and camouflaged to protect their identities, their circumstances are very real.

I have profound gratitude for the opportunity to not only create *The Coaching Forum* but to interact with readers when the columns were published. I got a lot of informal feedback about *The Coaching Forum*, especially when I attended national and international nursing meetings. Each comment was meaningful to me, and those conversations led to several pieces that were about readers' experiences, as told to me by the readers themselves.

Readers' feedback also led to the creation of this collection. When I decided to relinquish authorship of *The Coaching Forum*, a number of readers asked if I would compile a book of the many pieces I had written. Curating and narrating this collection has been a labor of love, and I am so grateful for their idea and for their continuing support.

Writing of any kind can be isolating, were it not for the lively and stimulating dialogues I have shared with my colleagues and friends during this project. I am lucky to belong to a thriving community of coaches within the Hudson Institute of Coaching Leadership Team and coaching community. I am also fortunate to be part of the Global Nursing Exchange, which convenes gatherings of nurse leaders whose commitment to collaboration is nourishing and palpable. I am also privileged to be part of the Berrett Koehler (BK) Authors' Cooperative, a spirited group of writers who are dedicated to producing books that promote a "world that works for all." Dr. Jesse Stoner, Dr. Marcia Reynolds, Dr. Beverly Kaye, Eileen McDargh, and Drs. Michelle and Dennis Reina are just a few of the BK writers who have become inspiring friends and colleagues.

I owe so much to the Elsevier team that carefully nurtured the idea of this collection from its inception. Yvonne Alexopoulos, my Elsevier editor, has cultivated the vision for this book as much as I have, despite her many other publishing commitments. She has partnered with me at every turn, sharing her expertise and opinions, always in the spirit of delivering what's best for the reader. Many others at Elsevier deserve mention, too—most notably Dawn Nahlen, the publisher of Elsevier's *Nurse Leader*, and Brooke Kannady, the production head for this collection.

Finally, I would be a far lonelier person were it not for my family and my friends, all of whom have supported this effort even when it meant I had to say no—over and over again—to gatherings, outings, and events. Thank you to everyone. Writing a book truly takes a village, and every person in my village has contributed to my well-being during this endeavor. Thank you.

TABLE OF CONTENTS

Knowing Who You Are as a Leader

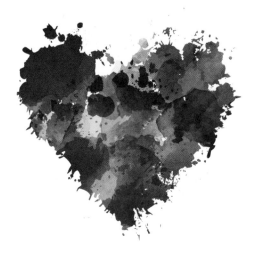

Leadership literature and our own experiences tell us that leaders who excel are those who know who they are. Masterful leaders are committed to being self-aware; they understand that they put their effectiveness in peril if they "self-forget" or are otherwise blind to their strengths, challenges, and impact.

Nurse leaders who thrive also know that self-management and self-care are among the cornerstones of their leadership prowess. They are mindful of their values, assets, and their learning opportunities, and they never forget what has heart and meaning for them.

1

The Stakes Are High, and You Must Change

What are you doing and who are you "being" as a leader? Think of crucial events in your professional and personal life, and remember what happened. Reflect on what you learned in those moments[a], focusing on what the experiences taught you about leadership.

Think back to a time when you faced a significant leadership challenge. It does not matter whether anyone else would consider this a crucial event. What *does* matter is how you experienced this moment in your life.

What comes to mind? Now, consider this question: *What important leadership lesson did this experience teach you?*

At this moment, if you are considering this question, you are engaging in the most important work a leader can do. You are reflecting on what you are doing and who you are being as a leader. You are harvesting the learning from your own leadership journey.

How often do we move from meeting to meeting, challenge to challenge, and task to task without examining our actions and the reactions they evoke? How often do we slow the action enough to ask ourselves if our behaviors are consistent with our values and beliefs?

In this piece, several esteemed nursing leaders offer powerful examples of just how beneficial this kind of reflection can be. To prepare for this column, I posed this same question to the members of the Nurse Leader editorial board. I asked them to share their stories and to consider what

they had learned about leadership. They offer two potent demonstrations of learning in action. These are not incidents others even noticed, but they are moments that literally changed these leaders' lives from that point forward.

The first case in point occurred in the start-up phase of a professional practice initiative. A crucial juncture arrived when this individual faced a compelling question: Was he going to stand up for what he said he believed about professional practice and allow it to be implemented? Or was he going to press ahead with his current practice of micro- and macro-managing every element of the process? How could he square his own behavior with the professional values he professed to hold? Was he going to take what he perceived to be a very big risk? Was he going to let go and allow others to step in and do their parts?

His answer was "yes," and with this "yes" came a highly successful program and "a pivotal moment in my own leadership and practice. It changed my professional life and pathway, forever," as he said.

Another editorial board member also spoke about an instance in which her beliefs about stewardship were called into question. She was frustrated because a decision had to be made about maintaining a costly program. The health system was facing financial pressure—continually—and this executive acutely felt the demands of keeping the costs down. She held a meeting with other senior leaders to discuss the fate of the program. After an hour of discussion in which no decision was reached, she announced to the group that she alone was going to make the decision.

Rather than accepting her proclamation, the team members pushed back. With respect, they told her that she had not allowed enough time for the conversation and that, although she was a participative leader, she was

---

[a]These questions are loosely based on an exercise that originally appeared in training materials for Kouzes and Posner's *The Leadership Challenge: How to Make Extraordinary Things Happen in Organizations*, Jossey-Bass. 1987–2017 (Sixth Edition). S.F., CA.

shouldering too much of the burden and the risk. What did this teach her? "That being alone at the top is part of the past and not the future. This totally changed my approach. From that point forward, I made far better decisions with the team. Equally important, I relaxed during my remaining 3 years in this position."

What do these executives have to teach us—you and me—about leadership? What common themes do their tales hold? In both circumstances, the leaders experienced a crisis of sorts, a moment in which they realized their behaviors were not working. The stakes were high. Their emotions were engaged. Notice, however, that their emotions were not hijacked. They were able to experience their feelings without being rendered ineffective by them.

Both of these leaders were willing to relinquish habits that had been in place for years. Each leader saw that times had changed. Their actions in these circumstances no longer served others or themselves. Both executives risked a new way of being. They were willing to evoke, listen to, and genuinely hear the wisdom others offered.

Each also faced a moment of fear—would the new approach work? With no guarantee, each said "yes," taking a substantial risk in the process. In summary, each of these leaders was willing to authentically and deeply change.

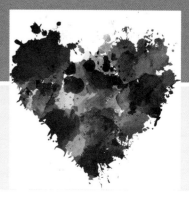

Practicing Radical Honesty

As leaders, we need to be unflinchingly real with our-
selves. We must reflect on how we are faring in our
roles and be honest about what is working and what
is not working. We must sort out our feelings, as well
as attend to what keeps us awake at night. We also
need to consider the meaning of the verbal and non-
verbal signals we give to and receive from others.

What do these facts tell us about our leadership?
Are you and I being the leaders we want to be? What
actions should we take to better align our day-to-
day behavior with the leadership vision we hold for
ourselves?

Why is it that sometimes learning sinks in and sometimes it doesn't? Many of us receive leadership training, and yet, despite our good intentions, we don't always integrate its lessons. We can speculate on why—heavy workload, excessive responsibility, insufficient support, etc. We can also take comfort in knowing that we are "doing our best" anyway.

However, if we're serious about transforming the way we lead, we can learn a lot from Della, a nurse leader who excels at changing her mind, emotional habits, and actions. Della is remarkable in her ability to "install" new leadership learning and alter subtle but significant self-sabotaging habits.

As her coach, I know that Della's success is hard won and unusual. Her story can teach and inspire us, especially when our professional well-being depends on making real and lasting change.

Della works in a community agency, and for the last year, she has spearheaded its signature community health programs. When we first met, Della was troubled and reserved. In private, she told me she did not feel understood by her boss or colleagues. She complained that she did not receive the support she needed, and she felt exhausted most of the time. She was apprehensive about her "fit" with the position. My three-way conversation with Della and her boss revealed that he too questioned her "fit." He confirmed that Della's colleagues were concerned as well.

Della had always been well-regarded professionally, so these comments deepened her uneasiness.

For the next few months, Della reflected on how she had presented herself at work. She dedicated herself to better understanding her behaviors and emotional tendencies when she is stressed. She became mindful of how she handles conflict, and she sought to comprehend her impact on others.

Della learned that she had subtle, reactive habits that damaged her relationships and chances for success in her role. She started to interrupt these habits and try out new behaviors; as she grew more accustomed to acting differently, she also became clear about the challenges she had been having on her job. Soon, after much discussion with her husband, even though she did not yet have a new job, Della resigned from her position.

TAKING CHARGE OF OUR EMOTIONAL TENDENCIES

The emphasis of this column is not Della's decision to leave. Instead, we are focused on how Della took charge of her emotional tendencies and "installed" new behavior, understanding, and self-awareness.

Della's first step was to become a keen and discerning observer of herself. For example, she realized she was endlessly replaying what her boss and her colleagues said to her. She discovered that when their "real-time" conversations ended, she continued the interactions "offline"—in other words, she kept talking with them in her head. There, she questioned what their words meant and whether they were telling her the truth. There, she concluded that they felt she could not succeed in her role.

Fortunately, Della became increasingly conscious of her one-sided replays and analyses, and she soon recognized that they were impacting nearly all of her work relationships.

She observed that her tendency to retreat into herself meant that she was no longer listening to or communicating with her colleagues. This withdrawal led to bruised relationships with the very people upon whom Della depended to achieve organizational goals.

As Della's self-awareness increased and the consequences of her reactive habits became apparent, she felt embarrassed and somewhat ashamed—at first. However, she learned to accept these feelings and allowed them to pass. She started to practice new behaviors and rebuild her self-trust. Eventually, she found fresh direction that buoyed her courage, confidence, and commitment to making emotional and behavioral change. These became the bases for her decision to leave her job even though she did not yet have a new position.

Here's *how* Della "installed" her new ways of being.

1. *She was honest with herself.* Della knew she wasn't at her best in this role. Despite feeling disheartened, she was able to take in her boss' feedback, receive input from her colleagues, and seek council from her own "gut."

2. *She was discerning about others' viewpoints.* Although she was open to her coworkers' thoughts and opinions, she did not take any of the feedback as "truth" on its face. Instead, she checked the "fit" of the comments. Were they entirely true? Were they somewhat true? If she thought they were not at all true, before dismissing them completely, she reflected on whether they contained even a small grain of accuracy.

3. *She worked hard to become conscious of her attitudes, emotional reactions, and internal conversations.* She tried to think and respond differently. When old behaviors resurfaced and she stumbled, she doubled her efforts to stop the old ways and practice the new ones. For example, if she was continuing conversations in her head, she stopped herself by simply saying, "STOP."

4. *She created a compelling "vision" for herself.* This was challenging, and it took several attempts; however, with time, Della formed a clear view of the kind of job she wanted to have. Her new vision became her basis for action—it was clear that the job in her vision was not the job she had.

5. *She valued her assets.* Della appreciated her ability to analyze problems, opportunities, and others' reactions. But she also realized that unchecked use of these strengths harmed her effectiveness and alienated her from her colleagues.

6. *She practiced being kind and patient with herself.* Della owned that she had given herself over to self-questioning and mounting insecurity. But by being compassionate with herself, she learned to spot and accept ill-serving leanings and stop them before they progressed.

7. *She elicited the support of others.* She talked more with her friends and trusted others. She engaged more frequently with her husband, and together they came to terms with their fears and concerns about their future.

Della's story is a compelling example of a leader who was willing to reevaluate the ways in which she conducted herself as a leader. Through diligence and a sincere commitment to change, Della "installed" new emotional habits and behaviors that will better serve her and those around her for many years to come.

3

You Are Not Happy. Now What?

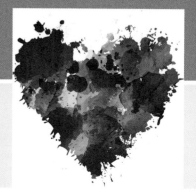

When the job isn't working for you and you're unhappy about it, it may be natural to look for something or someone to blame. Thriving leaders may start there, but they don't stop there. They have the courage and heart to discover precisely what factors are contributing to their disenchantment. They also ask whether and how they are adding to their own disillusionment. Then they ask themselves the hard question: Do they want to do the work to rectify problems and be masterful leaders in THIS role, or do they want to go somewhere else to make that commitment?

Imagine that you are a seasoned nurse leader and that you are stuck. You are bright and accomplished, but you are quite unhappy in your new job. You regularly receive calls from executive recruiters, so you know there is a good position for you elsewhere. After weeks of feeling unsure about your direction, you decide to seek executive coaching to sort out your thoughts.

In your early conversations with your coach, you complain that you are bored with your work and that you've had this and similar roles for two decades. You also say that your salary is lower than you could get somewhere else. In addition, you have problems with your fellow leaders. You feel that they are not as bright as you, and there is dissonance within your team because they don't "get" you.

If there have been times when you are not authentically committed to your work, perhaps you can identify with Lorraine's story. It is normal for talented human beings to fall into periods of disenchantment. What is not normal is to stay in these periods—to essentially take up residence in negative emotions and create more and better reasons to remain there, even though it is not healthy or productive.

When we find ourselves feeling off kilter, it is up to us to do what it takes to reconnect with a positive way of being in the professional world. We must make an effort to understand what is not working in our situation or ourselves, and we must be willing to change it. Contrary to what our first instincts may tell us, blaming others is usually not the right answer.

As Lorraine, an aspiring nurse leader, discovered, remaining negative can have a significant impact on our health, our work, and those around us. When she discussed things with her coach, she shared her conviction that "nobody at work knows how I feel," but she soon realized that this was not true; in fact, her disaffection was leaking in ways that were troubling and even dangerous. For example, when someone cut her off in traffic, Lorraine said she would "show them" by gunning the gas pedal to get back in front of the offender. Similarly, when she grew impatient with others on the job, she simply talked a lot or talked over people.

Although she was embarrassed to admit these things, Lorraine said that she was unable to stop herself from doing them. Even though she didn't like what she was seeing in herself, she had the courage to continue her exploration. Lorraine eventually came to a critical realization: her lack of engagement with the job she was hired to do was *her* problem. She began to deeply understand that she was doing a disservice to her organization, the exemplary leader who hired her, and herself.

This new awareness led Lorraine to a new question: what if she decided to stay right where she was? Even if she were to leave the job eventually, what if she refocused now and dedicated herself to doing the job she was hired to do—not halfway and not while simultaneously looking for another position? What if she really committed to doing *this* job as well as she could?

This is exactly what Lorraine did. This small moment became a major turning point in her evolution as a leader. The decision to fully commit to her work and this job grounded her, but it was just one of several actions that led Lorraine to greater success as a leader. Here are the others:

- *Lorraine actively observed herself at work.* She also solicited respected others' points of view about her strengths and challenges. She asked for feedback about the impact she had on people and how she contributed to dissonance with her colleagues when it occurred.

- *Lorraine was willing to take real risks so she could learn.* She took an emotional intelligence assessment that revealed her difficulty with allowing others to have their share of the credit. She learned that talking too much and providing information in every possible form were bids to elicit praise such as "you're right," "you're great," and, essentially, "we love you." She saw what was beneath her behavior: a need to feel superior to and admired by others to feel valuable and safe.
- *She was willing to be completely honest with herself.* She learned that hostile behaviors toward others were really strategies to self-soothe, strategies to make her feel better in the moment, even though she was sabotaging her relationships in the long run.
- *She was willing to let go of old stories and ways of being.* She realized that she had developed and needed many of these coping mechanisms when she was growing up. Many years ago, she had lived in an environment in which she felt she had to be on top to survive. While that may have been true then, it was not true now.
- *She was willing to be uncomfortable and to practice new behaviors even though there was no guarantee of success.* She tried listening more than speaking, and she did not habitually fill empty spaces with needless conversation. She showed empathy and compassion more than hostility when others were having difficulty. She felt calm and conveyed a sense of peace. She was willing to be humble and admit it when she did not have the answers.

Lorraine made a remarkable shift by simply changing her mind and having the courage to act differently. She focused on and committed to a deeper definition of what it means to go to work. After doing this, she said that working was much more enjoyable and that her colleagues noticed big and small differences in her behavior. They said that she showed much more trust and candor in her interactions with them, and eventually, by everyone's account, she achieved a huge win for her organization.

Lorraine's courage illustrates the importance of owning and addressing our dissatisfactions. Lorraine feels that her newfound and sweet success would not have been possible if the "old Lorraine" was still in charge. Fortunately, she grew tired of repeating old patterns and living in an old story. Now, instead of simply seeking a new job, she knows that the way she's always approached being out of sorts is not the best choice. Lorraine was able to change and shed her old skin, knowing it had served her in the past when she had to compete and win in order to survive.

4

Focusing Too Much on Other People

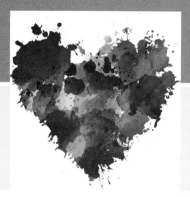

A measure of emotional intelligence is how much we focus on others and how much we focus on ourselves. Are we overly focused on everybody else's thoughts, wants, and needs? If so, what are the consequences of excessive focus "out there" and how can we shift the balance and reap the benefits of concentrating on ourselves too?

One of the most important ways to engage leaders as they grow is to focus on emotional intelligence (EQ). Management literature is replete with evidence of its impact, and it is my belief that we can significantly increase our EQ capacity with feedback, awareness, and practice.

As an executive coach, I work with various instruments that assess EQ, and I have noticed a trend in the results of some nurse leaders and managers. Their data suggest that they focus more on other people than on themselves, even though experts consider it "ideal" to focus on ourselves and on others in equal measure.

This does not suggest that the ideal is *excessive* focus on ourselves, nor does it imply that all nurse leaders are overly focused on other people. In fact, achieving an "ideal" balance is elusive for most leaders, and some nurse leaders do achieve good balance between these two perspectives. However, the trend toward focusing on other people is evident in the data I have collected, and this orientation can lead to undesirable outcomes. Here are two examples:

- Other-focused leaders may be out of touch with themselves, what they believe is most important, and the personal and professional values that could give them inspiration and ballast. Anchoring our stewardship in self-awareness gives us the clarity, courage, and strength we need to lead well on a daily basis, as I indicated in my book *Leading Valiantly in Healthcare.*[a]

- An even bigger consequence is that when we are leading and managing others, they rely on our direction, judgment, and lucidity. If we are not tuned into ourselves, it can be difficult to communicate convincingly and provide the clarity that others need to do well.

NOTICE THESE BEHAVIORS AND ATTITUDES

Here are some of the behaviors and attitudes that may indicate that we are focusing more on other people than on ourselves. Note that many of us behave in these ways occasionally. The consideration here is whether we feel or behave in these ways on a regular basis, regardless of the specifics of the situation.

- We pay more attention to others' wants and needs than to our own.
- Often, we do not know our own wants and needs.
- We put ourselves last.
- We don't have firm personal and/or professional boundaries. This can lead to over-functioning, such as finishing others' work for them, not holding others accountable, or both.
- We view what other people say, feel, or think as more important than what we say, feel, and think.
- We inflate our own value. This may not look like we're paying more attention to others, but it is possible that we may be "competing" with them in our own minds even when the context does not call for us to be competitive.
- We convey disproportionate anger or frustration that is surprising to others. They may not be expecting such an outsized reaction from us because, previously, we have not expressed our feelings. Perhaps, we don't know we are angry until our feelings boil over.
- We are excessively loyal to a boss, even when our weekends, evenings, early mornings, or vacations are frequently interrupted by the boss' needs and requests.
- We have difficulty saying no.

---

[a]Robinson-Walker, C. *Leading Valiantly in Healthcare*; Sigma Theta Tau, Indianapolis, IN. 2013.

- We want and/or insist that others agree with us because we seek their approval. Their opinion of us is more important than our opinion of ourselves.

None of these examples is taken from a textbook. Although they may seem harsh and overdrawn, these are real-life scenarios inspired by real nurse leaders and managers. If you relate to any of these, and you are concerned about your ability to shift gears and focus on yourself more often, here's what you can do.

- ***Stop and check in with what you are thinking, feeling, and wanting.*** For many of us, this can take a concerted effort, but with practice, we can become more aware of ourselves in any given moment in the day. It may help to remember that getting in touch with these basic aspects of yourself does not mean that you must act on this knowledge. One benefit of self-awareness is that you have more information, and you can decide to act on it or not act on it. Either way, you will make better choices as you engage in your work.
- ***Acknowledge yourself and your abilities frequently.*** Be aware of your capabilities and skills, access them when needed, and experience the appropriate level of ownership for the competence you have developed.
- ***Review your day at the end of it; remember and acknowledge yourself for what went well.*** Recall what didn't go well too, and think about how to avoid that outcome in the future. Consider whether greater self-focus would have helped.

- ***Breathe.*** Breathe again. It's easy to lose focus on ourselves, especially when we are challenged. Breathing returns us to our bodies.
- ***Be mindful of your role in a given situation.*** If it is to be the "doer," then by all means, get the work done. However, if your job is to oversee other people as they do the job, don't relinquish your role and take on theirs. Unless it is an emergency, consider whether your obligation is to supervise, coach, mentor, or precept. If it is, your colleagues will not learn if you forsake your role and do their work for them.
- ***Get feedback from trusted others.*** Do they see you as a strong leader or manager? If so, find out what they see as your strengths. If it's a mixed picture, find out how you can be more efficient, and notice whether more self-awareness will help.

Finally, catch yourself in the act of being more aware of others and less aware of yourself. When you find that you are focused outside yourself instead of relying on—or at least recognizing—your own thoughts, feelings, and wants, stop and redirect your attention. This may feel awkward at first, but it will probably not be noticeable to others. As you practice, it will become easier. Eventually, you can develop a seamless way of shifting your focus back and forth between what's happening around you and your internal experience. As you become more tuned into yourself, you will bring the benefits of your increased self-awareness to your leadership roles, your coworkers, and yourself.

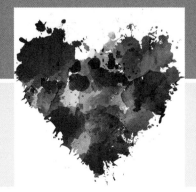

5

Taking Charge of Our Stories

When we serve as leaders, our stories are potent and impactful. The way we convey our message doesn't just transmit information, it actually creates reality for others—and for us. We profoundly affect others with what we say, and our words also affect our own emotions, beliefs, and actions. When we understand that we are the creators of our narratives and the decisions that result, we also see that we alone have the power to reshape them.

Joey is a young nurse manager with great potential. She is ambitious, learns quickly, and is willing to work hard to succeed. She is a relatively recent hire in her organization, having moved from another state with glowing recommendations from her former supervisor.

However, after a year on the job, Joey started having problems. She saw her position as too big, her colleagues as too undisciplined, and her boss as a poor leader. Meanwhile, her boss and colleagues experienced Joey as whiny, stubborn, and constantly blaming others. Her manager could see that Joey had the history and talent to become an excellent nurse leader, but he was not able to confront her directly about what she needed to do to get there. He was hoping that Joey's coaching would prompt her to change in positive ways.

At the outset of her coaching, Joey was eager to prove that she was right about her supervisor's meager leadership skills and her peers' unproductive work routines. Joey needed to tell her story and to be heard. After a few sessions of being listened to and validated for her positive qualities, Joey settled into an almost-shy vulnerability and a tentative willingness to share at a deeper level. She revealed that she strongly disliked her new town, and she was experiencing health issues and troubles in her personal relationships. Joey wanted to feel happier.

But how was Joey going to become happier? She was not interested in finding another job and moving, at least not yet. Eventually, as her coaching progressed, Joey started to look beyond her current conditions for the real issues that were creating her malaise. Deep down, she knew that her new circumstances were not perfect, but she had thrived in imperfect circumstances before. She could see that finding fault and trying to change other people, as well as working long hours to the detriment of her health and outside activities, were seductive habits. But they did not make her happier. In fact, they greatly contributed to her unhappy state.

The initial event that disrupted Joey's negative spiral was a test. She took a highly validated and reliable emotional intelligence assessment that is constructed to elicit real answers versus the answers we think we "should" give. Consequently, Joey's self-generated feedback offered her a brand-new lens to see what was going on inside her. Revealing and surprising as this fresh information was for Joey, it still would have been easy for her to dismiss it by blaming the assessment or the coach for her outcomes. But she didn't. Instead, she allowed the scores to resonate. She took them very seriously.

As profoundly impactful as her results were, it wasn't the assessment that disrupted Joey's unhealthy patterns. More important was the fact that she dropped her aggressive posture long enough to recognize the unvarnished truth. Much as it pained her, Joey admitted that the assessment reflections were accurate and that *she* was responsible for the deep unhappiness that she was experiencing in her life.

VALUING SELF-REFLECTION AND HONESTY

Shortly thereafter, Joey started a practice of self-reflection through journaling. She focused on being frank about what she was feeling and seeing in herself. She saw herself more clearly than she had for a very long time.

In choosing to be radically honest, Joey could understand how her behavior was harming herself and others. She made these admissions:

- She felt lonely on the job (and in the rest of her life). This was causing her to lash out and blame. The consequences were that she alienated others, and then she felt even more alone.

- She had refused to take any ownership for her part in the rifts she was having with her coworkers, boss, and others in her life.
- She had let languish her self-care practices, such as nurturing relationships with family and friends, and getting enough sleep and exercise.

Joey also realized that she could have a big hand in creating her own future by continuing to be scrupulously honest with herself. She could:

- *Recognize that she always has a choice in how she shows up,* no matter how perfect or imperfect other people may be.
- *Remember that she is in control of the stories she tells herself.* She and only she has the power to stop self-talk such as "I am a better leader than he is" or "I work harder than they do." Habits die hard, so when she unconsciously starts generating these tales again, she can train herself to notice what she's doing. She can remind herself that recycling these stories is unproductive and harmful, and she alone has the power to stop generating them.
- *Focus on small but influential ways to self-regulate,* such as pausing and breathing, instead of immediately reacting when something triggers her.
- *Rehearse by practicing new responses and behaviors* in upcoming difficult situations before they happen.
- *Acknowledge and concentrate on others' positive qualities and intentions.*

- *In challenging circumstances, learn new ways of communicating thoughts and feelings* clearly and directly, without blame and with kindness.
- *Find at least one trusted friend and/or colleague, who can observe, give direct feedback,* and help Joey remain truthful about herself.

Joey committed to holding herself to account as she goes forward. She also pledged to observe how she reacts when she is triggered. She will remember to breathe deeply, and if she forgets these things in stressful moments, she will keep practicing them until they become more routine.

She will also have a safety valve: if she doesn't measure up to her new standards, she won't beat herself up. Instead, she will forgive herself, be compassionate, and if appropriate, she will make amends to others. Most important, she will ask herself: what does this incident have to teach me?

Today, Joey says that she is a work in progress. As she continues in this job and advances in her career in this or another organization, Joey knows that her efforts will never be perfect. But she also knows that her behavior and feelings about herself will get better. She believes that eventually her relationships will improve and that others will notice that she is doing things differently, even if her progress is slow at first. She will remember that honesty and self-reflection are the keys to inspiring her will to change and to take action to make the change stick.

6

Being Accountable for a Leadership Mistake

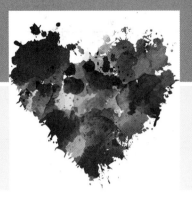

A good leader narrowly avoids an organizational catastrophe. What happened? How did she miss the signs of looming trouble? What did she do or not do that allowed the organization to come so close to peril? Instead of moving on to the next order of business after the danger was averted, this masterful leader chose to investigate and reflect on what occurred, and in the process, she learned an immensely valuable lesson.

How many of us "do right" by our leadership roles? By that I mean that we take our jobs seriously, we are sufficiently skilled, we take care of ourselves, we stay conscious of our values, and we attend to our own continuous learning. My long-time partnership with nurse leaders tells me that most of us do these things most of the time. We maintain a dedicated focus on professional excellence and goal achievement, self-care, and leadership growth. As health care professionals, we understand that these are critical components of our success and the success of those who we affect: our patients, colleagues, and staff.

So, how do we explain what some would call a significant "failure" when it is made by such a well-intended nurse leader? Phyllis is just this type of steward. She is devoted to doing her part to fulfill the organization's vision, and she understands and commits resources to ongoing learning and self-care for herself and the other members of her team.

Phyllis occupies a senior leadership role in a prominent health care system. She has held her position long enough to be adept at balancing the strategic and tactical requirements of her job. She has developed personal habits that enhance and support her capacity to focus, prioritize, and follow through. She nurtures her ability to set boundaries, to stay "on purpose," and to recognize what is most important in the short and long run. She also knows she cannot perform optimally without a well-trained team.

Like the rest of us, Phyllis is not perfect. The biggest trial she has faced throughout her career is her distaste for interpersonal conflict. Yet, as she has matured as a leader, she has endured numerous such struggles, including, but not limited to, staff performance challenges.

Phyllis still doesn't like these "conflicts," but she feels she has learned how to handle them well enough. When Tony, a key team member, showed signs of deteriorating performance, she carefully considered its likely cause before taking action.

She recalled that Tony had complained about family pressure, the scope of his responsibility, and his lack of sufficient resources to manage his function. Although Phyllis could not give Tony additional full-time equivalents, she did offer him extra staff help for a limited period of time. Additionally, she gave him more personal attention and support. Tony seemed to respond well; however, with time, his performance again slipped.

Phyllis decided to give him another chance, and once more, Tony appeared to do better. But soon enough, his performance flagged again. This time, Phyllis took more stringent measures to address the problem. With the help of human resources, she developed and implemented a formal performance plan. In the next few months, Phyllis felt relieved because Tony seemed to be improving in the ways specified in the plan.

However, something happened that upended Tony's progress. It was a big transgression with major adverse consequences. If Tony's mistake was aired publicly, it could have derailed the organization's strategy for the immediate future, and it would have had a grave effect on Phyllis' reputation and tenure.

Specifically, as Phyllis and the team were reviewing the final "blueprint" for an upcoming institutional meeting, she learned that Tony intended to offer wholly incorrect data during the gathering. When she confronted him, Tony claimed that the false information was a misunderstanding that was caused by others. But his professed innocence did not change the stark fact that he planned to deliberately deceive Phyllis and the entire organization. Had he proceeded, his report would have served as the inaccurate basis for approving the institution's largest project in the coming year.

After learning about Tony's indiscretion, Phyllis had a brief period of disbelief, anger, and embarrassment. Then, she and the rest of the team went into "fix-it" mode. Her organization's event was beginning in a matter of hours, and Tony's presentation was a big part of the meeting agenda.

Phyllis and the team quickly created a strategy for damage control, and they managed to run the meeting well enough to achieve most of their objectives. Simultaneously, Phyllis and the human resources staff dealt with Tony's errors, and he left the organization soon thereafter.

What is significant about this incident is that Phyllis did not understand what she did or didn't do that permitted this near-miss accident to occur. She is ashamed that it happened, and she wants to learn everything she can so that it never happens again.

Further details of Tony's actions are less important than the lessons this unfortunate event holds for all of us. Despite our own best efforts, we too may face serious mistakes that transpire or almost transpire on our watch. Whether the consequences are large or small, like Phyllis, we too can benefit from reflecting on our own unwitting contributions to preventable leadership errors.

WHAT BEHAVIOR DO YOU MODEL FOR OTHERS?

In this case, Phyllis reviewed how she conducted herself in the months that led up to this key organizational event. She thought about the pre-meeting preparation environment she and others created, the "health" of the team that was responsible for the meeting's success, how she managed Tony during this time, and what behavior she had modeled for him and others.

Here are some examples of the questions Phyllis contemplated:

- *Could I have prevented this situation by being less tolerant and more forceful with Tony earlier on?*
- *Did I have too much trust that Tony was following up with his responsibilities as he had promised?* Should I have been in "trust but verify" mode sooner?
- *Did the people around me know that Tony's performance challenges continued?* Did they see that he was faltering, and if so, what stopped them from telling me?
- *Because Tony's performance affected the entire team and organization, what other signs of trouble did I miss?*
- *Why did Tony intentionally cover up this mistake?* Did I and/or others do something to make it unsafe for him to tell us the truth? If so, what was it?
- *How can I align with the rest of the team to prevent similar problems from occurring in the future?*

These are just some of the questions that Phyllis considered. If you were in Phyllis' shoes, what else would you investigate? In the end, what would you conclude about the role you played in this unfortunate series of events?

7

"I Don't Have Time"

Time management isn't about time. It's about choice. It's about understanding and managing our priorities. It's about being aware of how we allocate our resources (including ourselves) on any given day. It's about understanding that when we hear ourselves say "I don't have time" we may be shielding ourselves from difficult choices that must be made.

Not long ago, I was invited to work with a group of distinguished nurse leaders from around the country. We were starting a year-long process that included individual executive coaching for each leader. As we discussed our upcoming work together, it became clear that many of these leaders had concerns about time. Some of them literally said, "I don't have time" for executive coaching or reflecting on their leadership.

I felt such empathy. How many of us say, "I don't have time" at least once a day? How many more times a day do we feel this way, even if we don't say it? Often our best efforts to manage time do not lead to the satisfying, well-balanced lives we envision. Instead, many of us feel frazzled and busier than ever.

Without intending to, some of us wear our "busy-ness" like badges of honor. We are so busy that we almost feel good about it, even if we have little time for our families and personal well-being. We come by our contradictions honestly. Being excessively busy is tolerated and even condoned in many organizations and in our achievement-driven society. Many Americans put a high value on "hard work," even when it is not healthy. Today's economic pressures can push us deeper into habits of working too much, often to the detriment of our personal lives. We are all trying to do more with less as

incomes decline and savings plummet. We feel that we have to be this busy because our financial pressures are real.

Most of us have the best intentions; we want to do a great job. To accomplish this, we have learned how to focus with aplomb. But what are the consequences when we focus like lasers and perpetually fill our calendars with more and more meetings and other "legitimate" demands on our time? Unfortunately, one consequence is that we become so good at focusing that we become blinded to great opportunities when they are right in front of us.

Some of us are so committed to our to-do lists that we do not see or hear new information that tells us that we need to shift priorities. We may not be as effective with others as we once were, but we can be blinded by the work instead of being open to the input that would allow us to adjust. We just can't see what we should see because we are so focused on getting it all done.

Some of us are actually addicted to our "busy-ness" and to being needed, even if this addiction empties other parts of our lives or causes colleagues and team members to over rely on us. Some of us are so busy because we don't delegate work as we should; some do delegate but become overly involved in implementing when that is no longer our concern. Why? Perhaps we feel others don't know enough about how to do it or they already have too much on *their* plates. All these reasons may be true, but they conceal the key question that we should ask ourselves as we plan our days: "What is the work that I alone can and should do?"

Many of us go along being overly busy for weeks, months, and even years with no discernable negative consequences. We excel in our jobs and sometimes in our personal lives. We may not feel as "happy" as we could be, but we are still fully participating in our lives. For some of us, unexpected circumstances force us to a hard stop and demand a steep price for our extreme dedication. If we haven't taken care of ourselves, we can become sick and require much care or rehabilitation. Or we can lose our jobs because we are no longer effective and because we did not see the signs when they started to appear. These and many other interruptions can temporarily or permanently suspend our "busy" and not optimally productive patterns.

HOW SHOULD YOU HANDLE YOUR MANY DEMANDS?

So what should we do? How do we manage our best intentions and the all-too-real demands of our professional lives? What solutions will give us a better quality of life and the biggest return, even if they require courage to implement?

- The first step is the most critical. *We must step back and away from the "I'm so busy" cycle long enough to evaluate what we are doing and why.* If we do not do this, the cycle will perpetuate itself indefinitely.
- *We must remember that we teach people how to treat us.* If we say yes too much, if we are available to handle whatever emerges, if we produce near-perfect results every time, we must realize that we are creating an expectation that we will always perform this way and that we will always do "whatever it takes."
- *We can identify situations that in fact do not require our self-imposed, unsustainable standards of perfection and excessive effort.*
- *We can engage in fundamental principles of time management, such as reexamining our priorities on a regular basis and recalibrating our areas of focus.* We can ask ourselves difficult questions such as "am I doing what is most important for me to do now?" "If not, why not?"
- *If we feel resistance to our own wisdom, and we know we need to shift gears, but we resist doing so, we must ask ourselves what it will take to change?* Being even more stressed? Getting sick? Having others view us with less regard? Losing an important relationship? Or can

we make needed shifts without such difficult personal sacrifices?

- *If we feel internal resistance to committing to what is most important, we must consider what else we are committed to that is preventing us from moving forward.* In other words, we must look at our own competing priorities. For example, is it more important to do almost perfect work when very good work will suffice most of the time? Is it more important to please others by saying yes when we really want to say no? Is it more important to feel needed than to allow others to grow into work that is theirs to do? Is it uncomfortable to face a life with more free time if we don't know how to fill it? Will we disappoint people if we have trained them to expect more of us? Do we know how to set new boundaries and explicitly adjust people's expectations in appropriate, professional ways?

WHAT IS YOUR BIGGEST TIME MANAGEMENT CHALLENGE?

Our biggest "time management" challenge is not managing the time in our days. It is managing ourselves. If we ask ourselves these questions and engage in these practices on a regular basis, we will find that our lives are more productive, less stressed, and more fulfilling.

The leaders in the room with me that day knew that they were at an important juncture. They realized that they were exhibiting classic symptoms of leaders who have become habitually too busy. How could they take advantage of this significant opportunity to grow if they were not available to receive it? They knew that time spent does not necessarily correlate with the quality of the results, and they saw the irony of their resistance.

Setting boundaries and creating new limits is challenging for the most courageous and skilled leaders, but these leaders were up to it. They knew—and we know—that such efforts can produce enormous benefits for others and for ourselves.

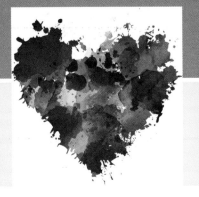

8

What Do You Choose to Animate?

Here, we look at the meaning of "animation" in our leadership lives. Animation means "bring to life." Animation in leadership is about focus—looking at what we are choosing to enliven as we create and talk about our leadership experience. Are we highlighting aspects of our work that are upbeat, honoring, and hopeful? Or are we emphasizing parts of our roles that are negative and outside of our control? What effect does our focus have on those around us? What effect does it have on us?

Like many of nurse leaders, Rich has too much to do.

He is a rural health system executive who leads managers and caregivers in a broad geographic area. Rich has been in his role for 16 months, and he has received consistently excellent evaluations from those above him. He enjoys working with his boss and peers, and he gets along well with his direct reports.

Lately, his organization's environment has been in flux, and Rich's priorities have expanded and changed. Although he understands the context of these shifts, Rich is frustrated and depressed. He is struggling to stay on top of his job, saying he simply "cannot get a handle" on it.

To make matters worse, Rich isn't eating right or getting enough exercise. So, he decided to get a check-up and seek advice from his doctor. Unfortunately, after his workup, his physician reinforced Rich's worry by painting a clear picture of the consequences of his poor health habits.

Rich came to coaching with a strong interest in turning things around professionally and personally, and his first task was to reflect on himself and his situation. He was willing to look beyond his immediate challenges, and he soon recognized that he is "hardwired" to take full responsibility for what needs to happen in all areas of his life. Rich wants to excel, and sometimes, he takes too much ownership, even when it is to his detriment.

Rich also cares too much about what other people think. He recognized that this can be a strength; however, he saw that there are significant down sides, too. For example,

Rich needs a great deal of external validation, and he frequently compares himself to others in the system, seeing their work as "more significant."

Rich noticed that he often focuses on what is lacking rather than what is working well at work. Rich is not alone; neuroscience validates that human beings have a natural negativity bias. Dr. Rick Hanson[a] calls this the "ancient circuitry" that homes in on what we perceive as threats. For some, this circuitry is attuned to what is wrong or missing. Because this predisposition is as old as humankind, it is up to us as evolving human beings to notice its impact on how we lead.

Rich acknowledged that he was focusing on the negative and setting himself up for poor emotional and physical health. He became more dedicated to finding and using better tools to manage himself, his work, and his life. He started by employing two self-management techniques that radically altered how he approached his job.

First, Rich recognized that his self-described inability to get a handle on his job was the result of factors that were beyond his control. Although he routinely negotiated deadlines and the like, it was simply not within his power to alter the scope of change that was affecting his entire health care system.

Second, Rich understood that he does have the power to respond to his challenges differently and more effectively. He realized that he was choosing to create and then "animate" many negative stories and feelings about his circumstances.

"To animate" means "to bring to life," and as leaders, what we bring to life summons our attention, interpretation of events, and emotions. To notice what we are "animating" is to pay attention to what we are enlivening with our valuable human energy. What aspects of our professional lives are we energizing? What about our personal lives? Are we expressing a genuinely positive outlook when

---

[a]Hanson R. Confronting the Negativity Bias. October 26, 2016. http://www.rickhanson.net/howyour-brain-makes-you-easily-intimidated. Accessed April 2017.

we talk about our responsibilities and commitments? Are we bringing the full measure of our presence and skill to the work that is on our plate? Or are we choosing to animate what is negative and lacking?

If we aren't sure what we're animating, we can find out by listening to ourselves and observing the narratives or "stories" we tell ourselves and others. If our stories are mostly downbeat, it's likely that we are animating discouraging descriptions and ill feelings.

Seeing and choosing what we are enlivening is not about ignoring conditions that are undesirable and within our power to control. Certainly, that which we can influence deserves our focus and best effort. But when we begin to pay attention to what we are animating, we may discover, as Rich did, that we are animating negative feelings and aspects of our lives over which we have little to no say.

Knowing what we are enlivening gives us the freedom to choose how we use our precious time and energy. As Rich discovered, the benefits of choosing differently are many, including increasing our chances of greater productivity and satisfaction. Rich realized how much time and energy he spent on speaking and feeling badly, comparing himself to other people and telling himself that his work mattered less than theirs. When he stepped back from these damaging stories, he was able to see and animate the value of his work and his many contributions to his health system's success.

Rich vowed to be mindful of what is and what is not in his control, and attend to what he does and does not animate. Consequently, Rich is well on his way to greatly improving the quality of his professional and personal life.

9

When Feedback Is Your Teacher

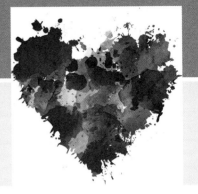

Feedback is a critical aspect of leadership development. Yet, receiving feedback is a big challenge for many. What is the value of candid, but critical feedback and what are some ways to manage it when it comes your way?

Kimberly was a successful service line director in a mid-sized medical center. The chief nursing officer (CNO) recently submitted her resignation after a lengthy tenure, and Kimberly was interested in her position. She had long felt that the CNO had retired on the job. Although the CNO was well liked in the organization, Kimberly was frustrated with her leadership, believing she herself was more qualified and ready to take over. As Kimberly saw it, she had successfully implemented many new initiatives, was well regarded within the hospital, and deserved to be the CNO. She was eager to roll up her sleeves and do whatever was necessary to obtain the job.

As Kimberly put together her plan to become CNO, it became clear that many factors would influence her fate, including how her peers, bosses, and direct reports viewed her achievements and personal qualities as a leader.

To begin, Kimberly created a detailed account of her accomplishments in the organization. Meanwhile, she also considered the potential challenges she could face. To learn what others thought and to discover any barriers they might present, she initiated confidential, "no holds barred" one-on-one conversations about her candidacy. She spoke with the CNO and others on her team, and she also met with other peers and people who reported to her.

Much to her surprise, Kimberly got mixed reviews about her CNO potential. Here are some of the comments:

- A few people said that she would be great in the role, but others gave only muted support.
- Some said that she excelled at service-line operations but that she was not a strategic thinker or player. Some people were uncertain about her ability to lead at the CNO level, particularly given the physician and community challenges the organization would face in the near future.
- She learned that some people had a decidedly negative view of her personal attitudes. They said that she complained a lot; several people said that they knew she didn't "like" the CNO and that her feelings created tension within the team.
- A number of her staff members no longer saw her as a "good" leader. This was a change. They said that Kimberly inspired and motivated them to do their best in the past, but of late, her behavior disappointed them. They thought that her attitude was negative and sarcastic.

This input gave Kimberly a considerable pause. She had accrued vacation time, so she decided to take 2 weeks off. She wanted to understand her colleagues' perspectives and she wanted the time to thoughtfully choose her next steps. For the moment, she kept her hat in the ring for the job.

During her time away, Kimberly asked herself many questions: What led to this feedback? If it was justified, what did she do to create these results? What were the most important steps to be for her to take now?

1. *She carefully evaluated the feedback* and considered how much and what part was accurate. Kimberly "checked the fit" of the comments. Were some of them warranted? All of them? None of them?

2. *She honestly assessed her attitudes and behaviors.* She knew that she in fact had become more vocal about the CNO and her certainty that she would do a much better job. Upon further consideration, Kimberly realized that she had shifted her attention away from her own leadership and toward her boss' shortcomings.

3. *She held her professional dream loosely.* She did not abandon it, but she did ask herself difficult questions. Did she really want to be the CNO? Why? What was this quest really about? If she didn't really want to be CNO, what *did* she want?

4. *She considered her deepest values.* She had loved managing the service line in the past. She loved leading

others, and when she could truly motivate them, it made her work all the more enjoyable and productive. As a team, they had accomplished so much. Now that team members no longer saw her as a leader they admired, she felt very disappointed.

5. *She realized that her emotions had been running the show.* Somewhere along the way, she had stopped paying attention to herself as a leader and instead started fixating on her boss.

6. *She questioned her need to be right.* Kimberly realized that she had let her sense of virtue and righteousness get in the way of her better judgment. Focusing outside of herself dulled Kimberly's ability to detect the signs that her key relationships were deteriorating.

7. *She thought about the skills she most wanted to emphasize going forward.* Kimberly knew that she was gifted at operations, also loved operations; she truly enjoyed creating and implementing complex plans for patient services.

By the time she returned, Kimberly felt renewed and refreshed. She was clear that she wanted to re-earn her team's respect and recommit to her current position and the work she really loved. On her first day of resuming, she thanked those whose candid comments were crucial to redirecting her attention to what mattered most.

Shortly thereafter, Kimberly learned that the organization had chosen its top three CNO candidates, and she was not among them. She was genuinely relieved. At the same time, she knew she had benefited from her potential candidacy. Her quest helped her reconnect with her deepest professional values. Her real dream was able to emerge. Kimberly's heartfelt wish was to be an inspiring service-line leader with a motivated team that accomplished great things for their patients. For Kimberly, this was more than enough for now.

10

Being Too Good

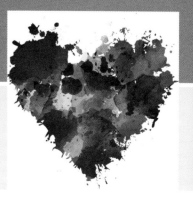

You over-function. So do many of us, and we wear our over-functioning like badges of honor. What are the consequences of functioning too well for too long? Are our organizations overly dependent on us and our extra effort? This cycle is unhealthy for us and those around us, so what can we do to reverse it?

Karin is a department head in a major metropolitan medical center, and she brings a wealth of unique and valuable experience to her position. She is about 2 years from retirement.

Karin elected to meet with me while I was working in another part of her hospital. We had about an hour together during which she laid out the everyday experience of her job. When she arrived, she looked upset and quite tired. As we talked, she veered toward tears several times. Karin described her work life as excessively stressful, demanding, and exhausting. She said that she had no time to think or plan and that she was working far too much. She described lengthy workdays and weekends in the hospital at least three times a month. With some pride, she said things had improved because she used to work every weekend.

When I asked her what prompted her to work so much, she cited several reasons, including uncertainty in the environment, concern about her personal finances, and the fact that her manager works this much. When I inquired further about her boss, she offered ample evidence that, indeed, the chief nursing officer seemed to work as much as or more than Karin. In Karin's mind, her manager's behavior sent her an unequivocal message: being on the job, this much was expected and not negotiable.

In my role, I encounter too many nurse leaders like Karin. They are well intended, good hearted, and genuine. Furthermore, leaders like Karin usually possess at least one of the following characteristics:

- They are very good at what they do. They excel in most or all of their areas of responsibility. Often, they also excel at the jobs they have left behind, the ones their direct reports are now supposed to accomplish.

- Whether they use this word or not, they feel like victims and believe that they are seriously overworked. They feel like they can't take vacations or go home at a reasonable time. For reasons that don't have anything to do with finances, they believe they cannot retire.
- They feel misunderstood. Their spouses, family members, or managers just don't understand that they don't have time to develop others or engage in self-care.
- Especially when they are very good at their jobs, they want things done their way. When direct reports and others don't comply, they cannot fully endorse their efforts.
- They have an exaggerated sense of their own importance.

THE SIDE EFFECTS OF BEING TOO GOOD

How many of us know—or are—well-intended nurse leaders like Karin? I suspect many of us recognize her, so it is important to consider the by-products of "being too good." Here are just a few:

- *We prevent others from developing their own abilities.* This creates dependence that harms our direct reports and us. This behavior inappropriately perpetuates newer leaders' tenure as beginners. For example, Karin said that she did not have time to train her three new direct reports. Two of them showed great potential, but they needed guidance from her. The third was already an expert but not in this new organization. She too needed Karin's thoughtful help.
- *We burn ourselves out.* We lessen our value because we are simply too tired to be effective. Sometimes we don't even know we have reached this state, and our colleagues can find it difficult to tell us.
- *We believe that we contribute to the success of our organizations because we over-function,* come in on weekends, and roll up our sleeves at every opportunity. But we don't understand that our over-the-top contributions can undermine our organization's capacity to create excellence by growing all its team members. We

inadvertently sabotage the system's long-term viability because we deprive it of filling its "bench" with robust leadership capability.

- *We model poor priority-setting skills.* We also model the inability to let go of responsibilities that are not essential for us to accomplish.

- *We fail to say no, over and over, showing a serious lack of personal awareness of our impact on others.* No matter how much we attempt to address, fix, and control the environment we are in, we cannot effectively manage it all. We must focus on what's most important and elicit the competent involvement of those around us for the rest.

- *We are unable to function within the boundaries of our roles.* When we do our work plus that of our direct reports, we are essentially condoning "over-functioning." If we are interested in developing a culture of accountability, we are sending the wrong message. Rather than encouraging accountability in others, our behavior creates passivity in others. By doing their work too, we essentially say, "Don't worry, I'll take care of it for you."

WHAT ARE THE REMEDIES?

So what are the antidotes for being too good? Even if leaders like Karin know they need to change, it can be very difficult to actually do it. Frequently, their identities and self-confidence are derived from achieving so much on the job.

If you find yourself in this scenario, or if you know of someone who is functioning in this way, here are some ideas to consider.

Karin has lost her ability to determine what's important. She is so accomplished and experienced that everyone in her unit depends upon her. Karin needs to take a hard look at what only she can do. Those—and only those—are the areas on which she needs to focus. She needs to create a plan to delegate more effectively or develop those to whom she already delegates. She needs to seek support from others to implement and sustain her new plan over time.

If we are too close to the work to see what the priorities really are, we need to ask for help to determine them. There are at least three sources of guidance available to us: the first and most obvious is the boss. Hopefully, this individual can step out of whatever benefit she derives from our over-functioning and into identifying the goals that are truly most important for us to achieve. Our direct reports may also be excellent sources of input. They know what they most want from us; they can see where we excel and the areas in which we have much to teach them. Let them tell us; we don't have to agree with all their suggestions, but we can at least listen. Finally, peers who work closely with us can also see our strengths and blind spots. They have good suggestions too. As with direct reports, we don't have to accept every idea, but we will learn if we pay attention.

If we are contemplating a very big change such as retirement or even moving to a different job or organization, and we are finding it difficult to move ahead, we can ask for help. We can seek support from our families, friends, or professional counselors or coaches. Major life changes such as retirement present enormous opportunities to grow and contribute in new ways. But for many of us who are used to organizational life, this next chapter can be difficult to imagine and even harder to initiate.

We can also ask for help from our bosses, direct reports, peers, and professional colleagues. If we are stuck in "being too good," and we sincerely want to change, we can solicit backing from those with whom we work. If we are genuinely committed to change, it will benefit not only those around us but us as well. Most people will be only too happy to work with us as we shift gears.

If we know we "should" stop behaving in these ways but are simply unable to do it, we can step back and away for a short time. We should ask ourselves what we really want in our lives. Is it an exhausting 60- to 80-hour work week? For most of us, the answer is no. But we may not have a clear picture of the life we'd rather have. Stepping away for an afternoon, a day, a weekend, or longer can give us the opportunity to carefully think about our next chapter. What do we want to be doing and with whom? How much do we want to work, and what do we want to do? What is our ideal day? What kind of contribution and/or legacy do we want to make? Answering these reflective questions helps us build out a vision for our own future. If we can become clear about this vision, we have a much better chance of creating it.

We all have something to gain when leaders know when to stop. Leadership that truly nurtures and inspires our organizations is that which focuses on self and other development. That allows us to serve well because we are personally "fit." We are in a far better position to attain organizational goals, superior patient care, and excellent customer satisfaction.

11

We CAN Manage Emotional Hijacks

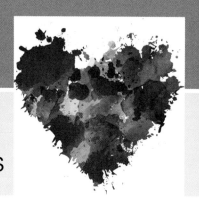

Most of us have the potential to be hijacked by our emotions. As masterful leaders, we need to be aware of our emotional triggers and sensitivities. We need to recognize when an emotional hijack is happening so that we can manage and be effective in spite of it.

Katie is a competent 40-year-old nurse manager in a Midwestern community hospital. She is sharp, well prepared, and committed to her organization's vision of quality patient care. In the past, she frequently suggested viable ways to achieve her unit's goals and resolve its problems. She made her recommendations even if they challenged the status quo.

Linda is a seasoned nurse leader in an academic medical center on the West Coast. She is a member of her hospital's top executive team and has received numerous honors for her achievements throughout her career. She is passionate about excellence in patient care and nursing leadership.

Each of these nurse leaders recently experienced challenging encounters that left them feeling off-center and vulnerable.

Katie described several meetings in which she perceived her boss' language and tone to be demeaning. She started to believe that her boss was marginalizing her or simply did not like her. Although she saw solutions to vexing unit problems, she stopped volunteering them because she thought they would be ignored. She felt angry and upset by behavior that she perceived as disrespectful and dismissive.

Linda had a similar internal experience. Although she had successfully interacted with the senior team for 2 years, she recently started meeting one-on-one with two of its strongest leaders. With both the vice presidents of human resources and finance, she reported feeling "tongue tied" and unable to confidently defend her

positions despite her well-documented facts. She even found it difficult to sit up straight and breathe properly during these meetings.

What do Linda and Katie have in common? They are way off their game. Both of these normally effective individuals perceive themselves to be weak and ineffectual. They cannot articulate their usually ready thoughts and solutions. Both have lost sight of and access to their considerable personal power.

Rather than leading with their competence, they are lost in negative, self-perpetuating reactive feelings. They are paying a big price. They feel invalidated, and they are acting that way too. Linda has stammered with both the finance and human resources heads. Katie has stopped speaking in group meetings in which her boss is present. Both Katie and Linda are out of touch with their professional focus and their effective presence.

These are normal human experiences. Katie and Linda are both responding to emotional triggers. The popular expert on emotional intelligence, Daniel Goleman, speaks about the amygdule, or the "reptilian brain." This is the seat of emotions that is hard-wired in humans; it is the home of the fight-or-flight response. We know we're reacting from the reptilian brain when our adrenalin is pumping, we cannot think straight, we lose sight of our longer-term goals, and we lose our sense of humor. Instead, we feel startled, afraid, angry, or intimidated. We are focused on fighting or getting away from the "perpetrator" of our negative experience.

As sentient beings, these and similar emotions mistakenly tell us that our very survival is threatened. In the heat of these moments, we can't see that we are reacting to our own emotional interpretation of others' behavior rather than the behavior itself.

The literature on emotional intelligence identifies two remedies for these difficult experiences. The first is to enhance self-awareness, and the second is to learn successful techniques for self-management. For example, to increase her self-awareness, Linda needed to step back and reflect on what she perceived as separate incidents of feeling ineffective with her colleagues. When she tried this, she realized that there was a pattern and that the behavior of both the leaders was similar—impersonal and standoffish. By contrast, Linda saw herself as warm and affectionate, but she viewed her colleagues as emotionally detached and disinterested in *her*. As she reflected on their actions, she realized that they behaved the same way with others. She realized that she was internalizing their actions and taking them personally.

Over time, Linda has gained awareness *in the moment* when she starts to feel powerless with these individuals. She has learned to manage herself differently by using a multi-step process. First, she offers compassion for herself rather than beating herself up. Next, she stops the action by taking a break. When she can, she suspends the conversation until later. If that was not possible, she says, "Let me think about this for a moment." If that is not possible, she takes several deep breaths.

When she implements her new techniques for self-awareness and management, she is able to detach and speak with confidence, even in the face of their behavior. She sees their actions for what they are—personality preferences that have nothing to do with her.

Katie had an equal challenge. Unchecked, her view of her boss' behaviors was eroding her confidence. As she became more self-aware, she began to witness her distress with her boss *as it occurred*. She decided to take hold and manage this negative experience.

First, she started to meditate each morning to increase her ability to stay centered throughout the day. As she grew calmer and gained self-control, Katie realized that she needed to confront her manager. When she did, she spoke honestly and directly. She described the behaviors that troubled her, she described the impact they had on her, and she asked her boss to provide her with direct, consistent, timely, and specific feedback about her work. In that session and a follow-up meeting, her boss appeared to listen and agreed to comply with Katie's requests. However, he did not follow through with his commitment.

Katie has reaped considerable benefit from her practice of meditation. Despite her boss's commitment to change, she has more difficult encounters with her boss. When they occurred, she was able to recover more quickly. She reminded herself that she was a competent professional and that her boss' unwillingness to give her specific feedback and follow through was not her fault.

Recently, Katie left her job for a new position. Although the unit lost a valued contributor, Katie made the right decision for herself. She used these unpleasant encounters as opportunities to grow, acquiring valuable self-management tools in the process.

Both Katie and Linda learned that every leader can be vulnerable and weakened when triggered emotionally. Both realized that the key to sustained leadership excellence is to be self-aware, compassionate with oneself, and, most important, a savvy manager of oneself. Our skill, our power, and our spirits are the most significant leadership resources we have. We must nurture them, and we must discipline ourselves so that we can enjoy and lead with the best of our competence, power, and presence.

12

The Destructive Power of Old Emotional Baggage

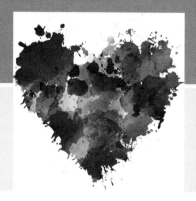

You know you need to stop the action when your plan for solving a management problem isn't working. If this unsuccessful strategy is the same one you've used and failed with earlier, why are you still using it? Is unresolved emotional business preventing you from changing your approach and adopting a fresh strategy? If you resonate with this question, read on to explore options for moving forward.

Not long ago I was working with Nell, a nurse leader who was challenged with managing one of her direct reports. Nell is a competent executive whose skill and expertise contribute mightily to her organization's success. But like all of us, Nell has vulnerabilities. One of them is that she is seriously tested when she must partner with a poorly performing coworker.

In this case, Nell was having trouble with Robert, a team member who needed to upgrade his results in several areas. His work affected everyone in the department, particularly Nell. But as his supervisor, she found it difficult to clearly articulate his improvement needs and create a corrective performance plan. Instead of working with him in a direct and objective manner, she hedged when they discussed what she wanted him to do differently. She set unclear objectives and established deadlines that were distant and loose.

Nell felt that she had a lot riding on how this situation turned out. She believed that if she couldn't turn Robert's work around, she would continue to suffer at the hand of his poor performance. She and the rest of her team would keep investing valuable time and energy in a relationship that was demanding too much from all of them.

Nell had access to human resources professionals, personnel procedures, and state-of-the-art performance practices such as objective behavioral feedback. However, these assets weren't enough. Why? Because Nell was unable to manage the consequences of her own unexamined feelings.

When Nell reflected, she realized that this struggle with Robert felt old and familiar, even though he was a relatively new hire. She had similar experiences with direct reports whose performance had frustrated her in the past. Because she was the more powerful partner, the direct report usually ended up either losing his job or being transferred. But Nell paid a price too. She had a bad reputation as a boss, and she knew it.

This story isn't just about Nell and her situation with Robert. Her circumstances are noteworthy because the cause of her challenge is common. How many times do we carry old stories, emotional residue, and lingering vulnerabilities into fresh interactions at work? When we do that, what is the quality of our presence in our professional partnerships? Are we able to fully participate when we are burdened with unresolved guilt, worry, or grudges? When such potent emotions are influencing us, especially in legitimately tough circumstances, are we able to engage productively? Can we bring the full measure of our expertise and objectivity to the table?

Unfinished emotional business can create serious blind spots for us at work. In Nell's story, we see that her awareness of her history and reputation is weighing heavily on her actions and capacity to think clearly. Consequently, she is inadvertently enabling Robert to perform poorly. She is dulling the requirement for him to improve by giving him vague guidance. Effectively, she is teaching him that inadequate performance is good enough.

Notice that Nell described their meetings as effortful for her and relaxed for Robert. This indicates that she is working much harder than he is, even though he has at least as much at stake. Another indication that she is working harder is her belief that she (alone) must be the one who turns this situation around. Paradoxically, by undermining Robert's capacity for improvement, she too is performing poorly.

SIDESTEPPING EMOTIONAL PITFALLS

So what can we do to avoid the emotional booby-trap that Nell unwittingly created for herself?

- *First, we can assess whether we have the skills, resources, and will to manage a perplexing situation.* Nell had both skills and resources, but she couldn't summon the will. She needed to find the reason; therefore, she explored her emotional responses and the limitations they were creating.

- *We can take on the uncomfortable task of being honest with ourselves when something we are doing is not working.* Nell knew that her ambiguous approach to correcting Robert's performance was backfiring, and she was courageous enough to admit it.

- *When we are challenged, we can consider whether our reactions are old, even when the circumstances are new.* Like Nell, we can look inside ourselves to determine whether familiar emotional patterns are influencing our approach to today's new demands.

- *We can face our own vulnerability—the one that is standing between us and a successful course of action.* In this case, Nell was afraid that her reputation would get worse. If she forthrightly addressed Robert's performance issues, there was a chance he would fail. If that happened, she would have to let him go and her reputation as a "bad boss" could intensify. But when she faced her fear, she saw that poorly supervising Robert was even more damaging to her coworkers' perceptions of her.

- *We can be clear about our roles and the boundaries of those roles.* It was not appropriate for Nell to take over Robert's stake in his own success and deprive him of accountability for the quality of his work. Yet that's exactly what she did by hedging on telling him what he needed to change.

- *We can be thoughtful about how we show respect for ourselves and others.* By allowing Robert to perform his job poorly, Nell was unconsciously dishonoring him and increasing the odds that he would be fired. She was also disrespecting the team and herself because they all had to fill in the gaps created by his subpar efforts.

Whenever we are burdened with potent, unexamined emotional baggage, we bring the effects of that extra weight into our interactions. When Nell chose to face and examine her "baggage," she set a courageous example for all of us. If she hadn't done this, she would have continued to engage in an unconscious "devil's bargain." She would accept Robert's substandard performance in exchange for minimizing future damage to her reputation. But she realized that in this "bargain," everyone was paying too much. So, instead, Nell made the difficult but appropriate choice to understand and manage her own feelings and their consequences.

13

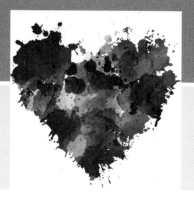

When Being Right Is Not Enough

A successful chief executive officer (CEO) is in an emotional slide because her colleagues are creating fissures in a key inter-organizational partnership. The CEO is angry and upset, and unless she intervenes (with herself), her emotional torque will grow and she will be unable to navigate the rocky road ahead. What can she do?

Lucy began our conversation sounding breathy and exasperated. As the senior staff leader of a large health care organization, she voiced her anxiety about an emerging conflict between her board of directors and another organization. She had other concerns too, but she was so emotional that she couldn't articulate them. After a little back and forth, she realized that she was also worried about having a serious conflict with her own board chairman. Although many readers of this collection do not have boards of directors, I hear regularly that you are presented with needs to "coach up" with your bosses. Lucy's situation is like many: her organization (or department or service) is at odds with another, her supervisor is taking an approach that Lucy doesn't agree with, and there are high stakes and big risks for both the organization and Lucy.

Lucy is smart, experienced, and savvy. She knows a lot about health care, the nursing profession, leadership, and her own role. Her story describes how she regained her power and leveraged her wisdom rather than being undone by her feelings.

As we talked further that day, Lucy said that several months earlier, she and the other organization's CEO, Sally, agreed on a strategy to address a mutual policy concern. This strategy required coordinated communications with their respective boards, staff, and constituents. Subsequently, Lucy found out that Sally had not proceeded as agreed. Lucy's own board chair conveyed this news to Lucy, and now her chair was crafting her organization's response. Lucy was very upset that Sally didn't do what she'd promised, but she was most upset that her own chair was orchestrating her organization's reaction.

Lucy had many questions. Why did Sally suddenly become an untrustworthy colleague? Was she exhibiting fresh-from-nowhere ethical or psychological problems? Did an external force cause Sally to change directions, such as her own board or a constituent? Why hadn't Sally communicated with Lucy?

Why was Lucy's board chair addressing both the policy issue and the breach of understanding between the two CEOs? Although the chair usually sought Lucy's opinions, why was the chair not asking for her involvement this time?

Lucy was very frustrated. She thought that neither Sally nor her board chair could see the folly of their ways; Sally had violated Lucy's trust and, with it, a critical inter-organizational agreement. Her chair was overstepping the boundaries of her role, acting almost as if she were the CEO instead of Lucy.

Lucy felt and sounded absolutely righteous. She said, "Every leader knows how important it is to keep agreements with trusted colleagues. Every leader also knows when to involve the staff, especially when they are the CEOs and in the best position to address what occurred in the first place." Wasn't Lucy due the respect of her position and the opportunity to clean up this violation?

So, what is likely to happen here? "Right," savvy, and focused as she may be, Lucy risks failing in this situation. Unless she makes a deliberate choice to slow down and examine her inner state, she may amplify her intense feelings and become even more caught up in circular, self-justifying thoughts. She will be too fused with her own feelings to consciously *choose* how to present herself and her ideas. She will miss the chance to use her considerable knowledge and experience to her greatest advantage. None of these outcomes is what she wants.

What can Lucy do to interrupt her speedy downhill emotional ride? First and most important, she must be aware of and validate her feelings, and she must stop herself from letting them escalate. She can acknowledge that she has every right to feel this way, but allowing her feelings to intensify will produce results that she does not want.

Once she stops the acceleration, Lucy can ask herself these and similar questions:
- *What short- and long-term organizational apprehensions does she have as a result of these events?*
- *What are her chief concerns about the actions of the board chair?*
- *Does she need more information? If so, what information?*
- *Who else can she consult to elicit respected and different points of view about this situation?*
- *Who is an advisor that Lucy trusts to provide her with thoughtful feedback?* In this case, Lucy's executive coach fills that role, but if she did not have a coach, who else could do this?
- *If Lucy were to successfully address her biggest concerns, what would her ideal outcomes look like?*
- *Given those ideal outcomes, what are Lucy's goals now?*
- *How can she mine her experience to achieve her goals?*
- *What specific action steps should Lucy undertake now?*
- *What help or other resources does she need?*
- *Will anything stop Lucy from moving ahead productively?* If so, what? How can she move through these barriers?

When Lucy asked herself these questions, she realized that she wanted to preserve and possibly deepen her relationship with her board chair. She remembered that she had been completely successful with handling an equally high-risk organizational crisis in the past. She recalled what she did and identified the skills she used then and how she could use them now. As her first action step, Lucy decided to ask the chair why she was not involved rather than discussing her feelings. Lucy mentally prepared to be as noncombative and as open as possible. She wanted to create the conditions for the board chair to speak honestly.

Lucy also recalled the considerable regard she had developed for Sally over their years of working together. She realized that she needed more information about what happened in Sally's organization that had influenced Sally so greatly.

Assuming Lucy and her chair could get onto the same page, Lucy would propose an interorganizational meeting to explore their mutual concerns, talk about their change of plans, and develop a plan for moving forward. The conversation could be CEO to CEO or a four-way meeting involving both the board chairs. To monitor herself in that meeting, Lucy would keep her focus on deep listening and her respect for Sally, especially when they discussed the breached agreement.

Lucy's experience offers us a gift. By all accounts, Lucy implemented her new plan successfully: the two organizations reached accord, and she deepened her working relationship with her board chair. Lucy's story provides a high-stakes, real-life example of a leader rapidly approaching the brink of poor stewardship because of an understandable but potentially unmonitored emotional hijack. Instead, Lucy exercised discipline, sought counsel, and created concrete ways to increase her understanding and regain her composure. Her reward was significant; she reopened her access to her hard-won wisdom, experience, and skill.

14

Manage Your Triggers and Find Peace

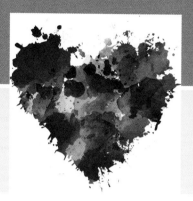

One of your colleagues is driving you crazy, and you know your craziness is as much about you as it is about your coworker. Can you see this relationship challenge differently? Can you shift from being judgmental about your colleague to being curious? You value your coworker's contributions, so how can you lead with your respect, courage, and values instead of your reactions? What would a win look like and what can you do to achieve it?

Casey is a nurse manager who enjoys and is fully committed to her profession. Like her peers, Casey has a lot of responsibility, and she does not take her duties or her career potential lightly. She has solid educational preparation and is proficient with the clinical aspects of her job.

Casey knows that courage, emotional skill, and maturity are also important components of successful leadership. So, when a recent exchange with one of her peers greatly upset her, she was eager to understand and learn from this incident. By Casey's account, the "triggering event" was serious enough to disturb her emotional equilibrium and peace of mind.

What happened seemed simple enough—one of Casey's colleagues, Jennifer, made some personal comments to Casey that she found disrespectful and condescending. Technically, they weren't human resources violations, but they were quite distressing for Casey. Although she wanted to "deal with it and move on," she was having a hard time doing that.

Instead, Casey found herself in an emotional quagmire that she described as following:
- She spent too much time experiencing "instant replays" of what Jennifer said to her.
- She had worked up a lot of anger and blame toward Jennifer. She was ashamed to say that she had also told stories about Jennifer to a few peers. Her tales concentrated on Jennifer's faults as a manager and as a person. Of course, she knew she shouldn't do this, but she did it anyway.

- She had persistent fantasies about what she would say to Jennifer if she "told her off."

Casey was embarrassed as she shared her predicament, and she was eager to find a healthy and productive way forward. She saw that she was in the midst of a self-perpetuating emotional drama, and she was acutely aware of the consequences of remaining there. For example:
- She was spending a lot of energy on these strong reactions, even though she was trying to act as if nothing was wrong. She was caught in an unpleasant cycle that was emotionally draining and distracting her from her work.
- Although Casey thought she was doing a decent job of keeping her personal angst under wraps, she questioned whether some of her coworkers sensed that something was wrong. If so, her colleagues would wonder what it was, and they would be curious and concerned. In the absence of hearing something from Casey, they would create their own "stories" about what was happening with her.

BENEFITING FROM A PAINFUL CHALLENGE

Casey knew that if she continued this behavior, her personal power and credibility could erode, and there could be lasting damage to the trusting relationships that she had worked hard to build. *This "learning opportunity" was painful for Casey, so here's what she did.*
- *She took a different approach to thinking about Jennifer, and she got curious about what it must be like to be her.* To Casey, Jennifer seemed lonely and needy, not just with her but with others too. When Casey considered Jennifer from this perspective, she felt some compassion for her. She also realized that Jennifer's behavior toward her was similar to the way she treated others. So, while Jennifer's conduct was not acceptable to Casey, she recognized that it was Jennifer's way of being with everyone.

- *These bits of compassion and insight were helpful, but they did not eliminate Casey's anger. She still blamed Jennifer, and she still wasn't able to move on. So, Casey turned her attention to herself.* She looked hard at her part in this difficult situation, wanting to better understand her own responses. She soon recognized that Jennifer's way of acting with Casey was evoking feelings that Casey had experienced before when she encountered condescending people.

- *This realization created even more motivation for Casey to diminish the power of this repeating pattern.* As an accomplished nurse manager with a bright future, Casey knew that this reactive pattern could negatively affect that future if she didn't address it now. After all, even if she could let go of what happened with Jennifer, there could well be other people that would elicit this same response. She needed to defuse these triggers once and for all.

Finally, Casey recalled how she had handled personally difficult situations in the past. She reflected on choices she made then, remembering that she had always taken "the high road." This meant that she elected to lead from her commitment to competence rather than from her lesser, more child-like self. Consequently, even in challenging encounters, Casey had spoken and acted with courtesy and professionalism. In the end, she always felt good about making that choice versus opting for the tempting lure of gossiping and holding onto grudges.

Casey eventually regained solid personal and professional footing with Jennifer and her peers. She chose not to confront Jennifer because she decided that Jennifer was "being herself" and nothing Casey said would change that. To Casey, this was a freeing decision that allowed her to treat Jennifer with courtesy, albeit with some distance.

Casey knows that her triggers will probably appear again. If they do, her predictable reactions may reappear too. But Casey is confident that they won't be as severe or as long lasting in the future. She may need more practice, but Casey is well on her way to maintaining her hard-won, treasured equanimity, even in challenging times.

15

A Compassionate Intervention

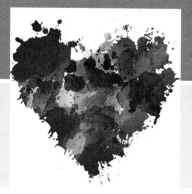

What does it mean to be kind to ourselves, especially if we "fail" and don't measure up to our own standards? Is self-care for a nurse leader "nice" but optional? Or is it a must for masterful leaders? Can we have compassion for and forgive ourselves when we have stumbled? What can we learn when we don't succeed, especially when we know better, and how can self-care and compassion help us grow?

When Bonnie first started working with me, she had just accepted a new nursing leadership role. She was young and excited about the opportunity, but she was also apprehensive about personal habits that could prevent her from being effective. After a few sessions, Bonnie identified the pattern that concerned her the most; she had a life-long "need" to orchestrate and control the actions of the others.

In Bonnie's new job, this tendency was showing up in the ways she treated her direct reports. She was hypercritical when they made mistakes, and despite her efforts to conceal her feelings, Bonnie showed her displeasure. She found herself jumping in and doing others' jobs when the better choice was to coach and guide. She was also having trouble articulating clear expectations without adding emotion—which usually came out as frustration and anger. For several months, Bonnie worked hard to understand the pattern and manage her feelings. Eventually, she let go of her urge to control and started to trust what her direct reports did. She also learned to enjoy her opportunities to mentor and inspire.

Bonnie evolved in these ways because she practiced and gave herself space to grow as a leader and as a person. For the next several years, she cultivated self-awareness and understanding, compassion for herself and others, and the capacity to notice but not be overcome by her initial reactions to challenging events. She repeatedly practiced new behaviors such as asking how she could help instead of simply taking over. Did Bonnie's dedication yield results? She would say, "definitely yes," and she can claim many examples of leadership success. She is especially happy about her recent promotion to a significant system-wide leadership role.

Still, Bonnie knows that her hard work is not over, and a recent experience drove the point home for her. When I saw her a few weeks ago, she was visibly distraught as she shared an incident that hijacked her new found skills and thrust her into taking over someone else's job.

As she told her story, she realized that, although quite taxing, the circumstances did not constitute an emergency, and her direct report could have managed the situation perfectly well. Yet, Bonnie interfered and behaved just as she would have many years earlier. What was the issue? Had Bonnie's considerable investment in her own growth not taken hold? Did she have a relapse from which she could not recover?

After sharing the details, Bonnie developed the beneficial perspective of hindsight. She saw that, in fact, perplexing conditions like these happen all the time in nursing leadership, and that her ill-serving behavior was not spawned by the specific circumstances. The triggers instead lay in Bonnie herself. When this event happened, she was overly tired and she had allowed herself to be spread far too thin. As a result, she was especially susceptible to feeling pressured, anxious, and frightened.

Today, Bonnie is the first to say that the happenings on that day did not have to hijack her feelings and dictate actions she would regret. She also accepts that no matter how much she has practiced, poor self-care can quickly return her—and any of us—to old habits.

Once she recognized this very human tendency, Bonnie decided to put an easy-to-remember plan in place. She likes to think of it as a "compassionate intervention" with herself. Here is what Bonnie resolved to do if (and when) she is not at her best and similar events happen again.

1. ***She will stay alert and notice when she is focusing on others' wrongdoings and/or fixing their problems.*** Instead of allowing that dynamic to continue, she will redirect her attention back to herself.

2. ***She will stop the action and pause long enough to breathe.*** Then she will use a mindfulness technique: she will temporarily suspend whatever story she is telling herself about the situation and the people involved. She will simply let it go; she will not reprimand or try to talk herself out of her narrative. She will just set it aside for a moment.

3. ***Then she will turn her attention to what she is feeling.*** She will be patient as she identifies the sentiments that have been triggered. For example, she could feel fearful, victimized, shamed, or worried about looking bad or incompetent. Or, she may feel unappreciated and unheard, especially if she has spent time mentoring those around her.

4. ***Once she has identified the feelings, she will be in a better position to move forward in a less reactive way.***

Taking these steps requires only one thing—Bonnie must remember to pause before acting on her feelings when she is particularly vulnerable to pressure and stress. Initiating her simple plan will give her room to breathe and remember who she is now as a leader. She will once again have access to the new behaviors she has practiced many times. Most important, she will be able to return herself to a state of emotional balance and right action.

Whether we are new to leadership and management or have been in the role for many years, all of us can be emotionally hijacked. When we are tired and spread too thin, even the most experienced among us can be quickly transported to raw and immature responses.

Bonnie reminds us of our most potent tools in taxing times: to slow down and breathe and turn our attention away from our story. Taking just these two steps allows us to return our focus to ourselves, and understand and redirect what is happening emotionally. No matter how long we have served as leaders, all of us can choose to interrupt our own reactions when we know they will do more harm than good.

Establishing Healthy Boundaries

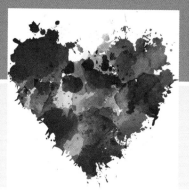

Self-care is about more than days at the spa and relaxing at home. It is about courageous action that is based on self-regard and self-responsibility. From these values comes a particularly important example of self-care—a masterful leader's ability to establish healthy boundaries. Healthy boundaries include ways in which we honor, yet do not take on, the work and problems of others. Healthy boundaries also include treating ourselves in ways that leave us feeling inspired, refueled, and ready for the leadership work that's ahead.

Charlotte is a nurse leader who is concerned about the attitudes of the leaders and managers who report to her. She readily admits that they have weathered significant organizational changes in the last year, and she praises them for their efforts to absorb the transitions while continuing to provide excellent patient care.

Her concern has to do with the team's poor morale. Here are some examples:

- Even though the organization has provided resources and assistance to help them through the significant transitions that have occurred, they blame others for their circumstances.
- Some are dissatisfied with their jobs, but they are not initiating constructive conversations with those who can hear them out and help them adjust the job or change positions.
- A number of them are overly focused on what other people think and (apparently) feel about them.
- They speak like victims, making statements like "I was thrown into this role," even though their role changes occurred more than a year ago.
- When they hear their peers complain inside conversations, they join in and inadvertently amplify their problems. They do this in spite of Charlotte's encouragement to publicly speak up and voice their concerns so that they can be addressed.

The focus of this column is not on what Charlotte can do differently, but what her team members can do differently to help themselves and the organization, regardless of what senior leadership does or does not do.

What each of these leaders can do is pay close attention to their own boundaries. We sometimes think that healthy boundaries mean that we appropriately differentiate between ourselves and other people, but healthy boundaries are also about how we treat ourselves. No matter how evolved our organizations are, it will always be up to us to pay attention to and support our own emotional health and well-being.

As leaders, none of us can afford to wait for someone else to take care of us and then blame them when they don't. This may seem obvious, but when leaders perpetually engage in victim-like conversation and behaviors, they are giving away their professional and personal power. In effect, they are turning over their emotional health on the job to others. This is a mistake. When we are professionals, other people are not and cannot be in charge of our self-respect and sense of well-being.

BOUNDARIES AND SELF-RESPECT

But what do the concepts of self-respect and well-being really mean when it comes to establishing boundaries that keep us well and whole at work? Here are some tips:

- ***Think about what self-respect and self-kindness mean for you.*** Many of us use the word "respect" when it comes to other people, but we are not always clear about the behaviors involved. In what ways do we demonstrate respect and kindness for others? Are those the same ways in which we demonstrate kindness and respect for ourselves? What are some specific examples of times in which you have been kind to yourself at work? How do you feel about yourself when you respect yourself in those ways?
- ***Practicing healthy boundaries means that we remember and own our part in our problems and challenges.*** This isn't easy. But it's empowering when we realize that

we may have some slice of responsibility, however small, for an outcome that isn't to our liking. Identifying our part takes us out of blaming others (and disempowering ourselves) and puts us in a position to do something about what's not working for us.

- *Doing something about what is not working for us often means speaking up.* This contrasts with arguing our points to our friends or recycling our complaints and bad feelings inside our own heads. When we neglect to say anything to those who can and should be aware of our concerns, we are not taking care of ourselves. Speaking up effectively means knowing our wants and our needs and being able to articulate a rationale that's appropriate for our organizational environment. It also means attending to the emotions that accompany what isn't working for us. Speaking up effectively may require "rehearsals," and if that's true for you, you're in good company. Many excellent leaders practice their words with trusted others in private before saying them "for real" when the stakes are high. Knowing how to name, honor, and express our feelings clearly and unemotionally is part of managing our boundaries and empowering ourselves.

- *There are times when we are, in fact, "blameless" for circumstances that affect us greatly. Those are the situations in which we have no control.* In such cases, what is our responsibility for moving forward in a way that is healthy for us and for those around us? How can we honor our emotions, upset as we may be, without having them upend our effectiveness as leaders and caregivers? What does self-respect look like in that case? Each of us has our own answers to these questions. What are yours?

- *Self-awareness and reflection can help us strengthen our boundaries.* Being cognizant of how much we focus on the opinions, actions, and feelings of other people gives us a clue as to whether we are overly focused on everybody else. Pulling some of that attention away from them and putting it onto ourselves permits us to know and value our own viewpoints as much as those of others. Doing this can help restore our well-being and self-respect.

In the end, Charlotte supported her team as they learned about, practiced, and eventually took on more ways of exhibiting healthy boundaries toward each other, the organization, and, most importantly, themselves. They realized that allowing their own power to "leak" by blaming others, the institution, and the past was hurting themselves more than anyone else. Most important, they realized that they–and only they–were responsible for their own happiness on the job.

17

When Good Intentions Go Awry

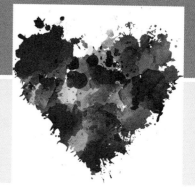

"That of which we are unaware owns us."[a] Sometimes, we work too much and we over-attend. When we do this too often, many of us let go of self-care and put ourselves at risk. Doing too much at the expense of our health and well-being could mean that we are no longer fit for our leadership roles. At the very least, we are not as fit as we could be, so it is easier to become overwhelmed and blind to important cues about our organization's, and our own, most significant needs.

We usually think of a strong commitment to work as a positive attribute for leaders, but this column offers a story of two nurse leaders whose intense dedication actually hurt their performance, rendering them ineffective.

Martha is a nurse leader in a large national organization, and she is experiencing a great deal of difficulty in her new role. She has angry outbursts with colleagues, and she does not see eye to eye with the chief executive officer (CEO). She believes that another member of the senior team is "out to get her," and she has examples that "prove" this. Although her CEO still hopes that Martha will succeed in her role, he has insisted that she retain an executive coach to give her a boost.

Gloria is the CEO of a complex health care organization, and she too is having trouble on the job. Unlike Martha, Gloria has been in her role for many years. Gradually, she has grown frustrated with the board of directors. Despite her consistent efforts to offer "a better way," the board is moving the organization forward in ways that she does not completely support.

Lately, Gloria's frustration has grown. At the same time, the board has registered concerns about her performance. Gloria feels defeated and angry, and her dialogues with the board are increasingly at odds. Her usually full schedule has become even more demanding. She says that she is "too busy" to exercise and often eats heavy meals. She

has difficulty sleeping without medication. Her limited free time is consumed with chores, and she does not have time for her children and grandchildren.

Although Gloria and Martha lead very different health care entities, they share important characteristics:
- They are highly educated and experienced nurse leaders.
- Their work in the health care world has brought them respect, acclaim, and recognition.
- Until now, they have been effective and persuasive in their roles.
- They are both on the precipice of abruptly leaving their jobs, either because they can't tolerate the conditions or because they will be fired.
- There is a victim-like quality in their descriptions of their predicaments.
  What else do Gloria and Martha have in common?
- Neither is taking care of herself. Gloria's self-care habits are compromising her efficacy and possibly her long-term health. Martha has had life-long medical challenges that, with attention, can be accommodated in a busy professional's life. Indeed, Martha has successfully managed them for years until now.
- Neither can see her own resistance and the impact of that resistance on the powers that be. One is resisting the board, and the other is resisting the CEO and other senior staff. Neither comprehends that her resistance is negatively affecting her behavior and performance.
- Neither can see that she is overwrought and that her ways of "giving" on the job and "staying the course" are producing diminishing returns. The ways in which these leaders are demonstrating their commitments are actually hurting their effectiveness, and not just a little bit.
- Each has been given clear feedback that her performance is not optimal: Gloria has received less-than-glowing performance reviews, and Martha's CEO insisted that she see a coach for corrective help. Despite this irrefutable evidence, both leaders continue to bring the same behavior and viewpoint to their work.

---

[a]Peter Hawkins (Advanced Coach Seminar; The Hudson Institute of Coaching, April 11, 2019).

Before we conclude that these leaders are anomalies with possible emotional or mental difficulties, it is important to consider their positive attributes and intentions. One started her new job by immersing herself in learning. She devoted many nights and weekends to understanding everything she could about her new role. Unfortunately, her positive intentions led to doing too much, and this compromised her health just as she began to grapple with the politics of her new position.

The other is a strong leader and an expert in her field. She knows she has a lot to offer; it is very difficult for her to relinquish the authority she believes she has earned, particularly when there are board members who know far less than her.

What should these leaders do to reverse course and recapture control of their own futures? Their best options are surprisingly simple, and most involve self-care. We think of self-care as so obvious that its value is easily understated. We ignore self-care and its importance at our own peril, however. Without enough rest and time away from the intense work of leadership, Gloria and Martha are rendered blind to what is right in front of them: they are not effective and their coworkers are telling them this in no uncertain terms.

Other remedies are also critical and not so easy.
- *Each leader's resistance can be her teacher.* When we are leading and people resist us, it behooves us to examine the feedback to see if there is a modicum (or a lot) of "truth" in the complaint. When we ourselves resist, it is wise to acknowledge and examine our own resistance to see what truth our feelings may contain. For example, Martha accepted her new position without a full understanding of its challenges. Her eventual resistance was a reaction to being exhausted and not being perceived as competent for the first time in her professional life. Gloria resisted a negative performance appraisal when she felt she knew more than her board and had done everything "right." Her weariness precluded her from seeing her own attitude and its effects. Her diminished physical state prohibited her from acknowledging the board's legitimate right (and obligation) to guide the organization as it saw fit.
- *When people question our leadership performance, it is important to consider what is being said.* Wise leaders

are aware of their emotional state (tired, frazzled, feeling like we can't win, etc.) and acknowledge resulting tendencies such as blaming others. Refreshed leaders know that only they can redirect what is happening to them and thoughtfully navigate the best ways forward.

WHERE DO MARTHA AND GLORIA GO FROM HERE?

First, Martha can ask herself whether she really wants this job. The cost to her family and herself is considerable. She may not want to admit that her choice was a mistake, but it is preferable to acknowledge that rather than to sacrifice her health, her family's well-being, and her reputation.

If Martha does want this job, can she work less and establish better health habits? Is she willing to discipline herself and eat properly, exercise enough, and get sufficient sleep? What will it take for her to make this level of commitment to herself and her own care?

Is Martha willing to do what it takes to re-engage with her colleagues? Can she openly listen and adjust her style and her work products to meet the CEO's expectations? Is she willing to do the hard work of addressing her challenges with the fellow leader who is "out to get her"?

Gloria has a different set of decisions. She has been in her role for a long time, and the board of directors has been pursuing a course that she does not favor. The board shows no signs of shifting. Gloria needs to consider whether this position is still the best fit for her.

If she decides she still wants to be in this job, what will it take for her to fully support the board's decisions? Can she direct the staff and guide the resources of the organization so they accelerate the mandates of the board? Can she authentically embrace the board's goals and expectations?

Both leaders need to let go of what they believe to be past injustices. Can they do this? In what ways can they reframe past events so they no longer see themselves as victims? Can they let go of the wrongs they feel have been done "to" them?

Although Martha and Gloria's stories may be different from your own, their journeys vividly illustrate the dangers of excessive good intentions, hard work, and long hours when the fruits of so much labor are not what we expect.

18

What Learning "Spirals" Teach Us

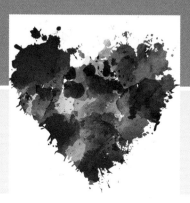

When we grow as leaders, we learn valuable lessons about how to be more effective. Sometimes those same "learning opportunities" come back again later in a new form. They return because installing real learning and change can take a great deal of time, practice, and patience. It is our job to give ourselves that time, sometimes a lot of time, and offer ourselves compassion when we don't change as fast as we would like.

What type of a learner are you? When you are being educated about leadership, do you take in knowledge quickly? Do you easily incorporate new information and practices into your routine? Or do you learn more gradually, encountering key teachings more than once and absorbing them slowly over time?

Or, perhaps are you like Wanda, a leader who learns in both ways? Wanda is a well-regarded nurse executive who is polished, articulate, and dedicated to the well-being of her organization's patients. She has received numerous professional acknowledgments throughout her career.

As her coaching partner, I know Wanda has faced steep challenges, and I have seen her handle them with aplomb, at least on the outside. But we have both noticed something else: the players and the details change, but at their core, her biggest obstacles are almost always about the same thing. Wanda and I call these repeating themes her "learning spirals." Each time she meets a "lesson," yet again she pauses to think deeply about what has happened and why.

Initially, Wanda found these "spirals" frustrating, wondering why she couldn't just "get it" the first time. Eventually, she understood and forgave herself for her human propensity to go through significant leadership "tests" more than once or even many times. Now, when she goes through a learning spiral, she has a fresh view of its impacts, and she has more tools to combat its potency.

Let's get specific. One of Wanda's greatest challenges is her desire to be liked. Early in our partnership, Wanda realized that she not only wanted to be liked, she *needed* to be liked. She had an intense longing for validation and acknowledgment from others. Although she received lots of accolades from her colleagues, they never seemed to satisfy her.

Left unconscious and unchecked, the consequences of Wanda's need for approval severely affected her leadership and the quality of her life. A few ramifications were:

- Wanda had great difficulty saying "no." So, she almost always said "yes" to requests, thereby losing control of her time. Consequently, she lost any semblance of balance between her personal and professional life, and she privately complained of being overworked and tired.
- When Wanda was recognized for her contributions, she did not take others' appreciation to heart. She was outwardly gracious, but inside she was "shy," deflecting even the most heartfelt acknowledgments.
- Her need for acclaim also affected her marriage. Her husband had problems of his own, and when he failed to provide continuous positive reinforcement, Wanda felt unseen and unheard, even though she knew he loved her very much.

LESSENNING THE GRIP OF OUR LEARNING CHALLENGES

Once Wanda clearly saw her long-held requirement for recognition, she took steps to reduce its power:

- ***She practiced saying "no" even when it was uncomfortable.*** Instead of reflexively allowing herself to say yes so she could "help," she thought carefully about each request. Was it a priority for her, her team, or her organization? If not, could she genuinely afford the time and effort it would take? She also thought about whether someone else was better equipped to take on the responsibility. How could she delegate more and provide others new opportunities to develop and grow?
- ***She reflected on why she needed so much external approval.*** She thought about her professional and personal recognition, seeing again that no matter how much

there was, it was never enough. This process took time, but eventually she accepted that the recognition she sought from others would never satisfy her. Eventually, she realized that what would help her most was genuine self-love and gratitude. She began a daily practice of acknowledging the many gifts and joys that existed in the life she had built. Most important, she started to genuinely value the role she was playing in her own success.

- *She regularly reviewed her priorities at work, at least weekly and sometimes more often.* This practice kept her focused on what was most important and discouraged her participation in nonessential activities.
- *She asked a trusted colleague to help her concentrate on her priorities and her new found practice of saying "no."*

Wanda was successful in seeing herself through new eyes and incorporating new behaviors that enhanced her well-being, both on and off the job. However, a few months later, she encountered another situation in which she said yes to a low-priority, time-consuming request even though she was swamped with work. Once again, she had given in to her strong need to be liked.

So, what happened? Had Wanda forgotten her increased self-awareness and hard-won growth? No. Wanda remained dedicated to improving her leadership. But Wanda is like many of us who make fundamental changes in how we interact with the world: we fall backward from time to time. Changing deep-seated habits takes time, sometimes a long time.

As Wanda thought about this "slip," she appreciated that needing to be liked was a life-long pattern. It's not easy to override, but she also respected that she had built a "tool chest" of ways to remain motivated.

Now, many months later, Wanda recognizes that her "like me" need comes up again and again. Usually, she takes a breath and chooses how she will respond. But if she does slip, she reminds herself that profound learning and abiding change can take many years. She also remembers that her new behaviors will eventually become habits too.

Wanda is on the path to a greater personal and professional satisfaction. Along the way, she is embracing new strategies to stay on plan:

- When the old reflexive behavior comes up, she sees and manages it more quickly.
- She (quietly) celebrates when she stops short of saying "yes" without thinking.
- She finds new ways to affirm what she does well and who she is as a person and as a leader.
- She no longer brushes off acknowledgments she receives. Instead, she savors them.
- She reminds herself of the consequences of falling back into habitually saying "yes."

Wanda's growth as a leader is a work in progress. Still, she knows that her learning spirals contribute to a fulfilling journey that is well worth taking.

Building Relationships That Thrive

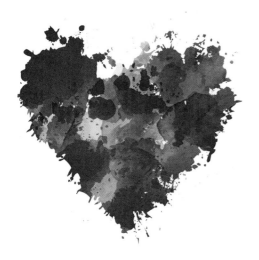

Nurse leaders who thrive have an array of relationship strategies for the good and the bad days. They are skilled at influencing and managing their expectations of others, and they know how to manage their disappointments in others too. They know how to avoid interpersonal "traps" by building on their self-awareness, values, communication skills, and ability to focus. They thrive by bringing the best of themselves to their key relationships on (and off) the job.

19

Passion Two Ways

You're passionate. You are a Healer who pays attention to what has heart and meaning, and you are a champion for quality patient care. Do you communicate your values and share your zeal in ways that inspire others? Or is it possible that, at times, your strongly held convictions prevent you from being open to and valuing the opinions of other important stakeholders? How can you convey your fervent point of view respectfully, without shutting colleagues down?

This is a story of two leaders who are passionate about the health of their patients. They are equally passionate about nursing and its importance in nearly every aspect of health care delivery today.

The first leader, Hannah, is a successful vice president in a large metropolitan medical center. Hannah has a challenging role that is vital to the health system's short- and long-term goals. To achieve these goals, she must successfully enlist the support and voluntary participation of many stakeholders throughout the organization. Hannah has neither a large budget nor direct authority over the many physicians and others she must recruit for her programs.

Hannah is not an extrovert by nature, but her single-minded focus, her clarity about her role, and her enduring passion enable her to recruit all the personnel she needs for her programs. By every measure, Hannah is very successful in her job.

The second leader, Celeste, is also a nurse leader who champions the importance of patient care and nursing's role in providing it. She too is a well-educated, accomplished vice president in a medical center.

In her current job, Celeste must also educate and motivate her colleagues. Successful execution of her responsibilities relies on her ability to influence health care professionals inside and outside the medical center. She too has an obligation to advance the organization's mission and vision in innovative ways. However, at times, outside of nursing circles and her direct reports, Celeste does not feel she is effective in promoting her ideas. In candid moments, Celeste says she knows that people stop listening to her after a while. Her usual response is to get upset and "go all out" to try to convince others of the virtue of her cause. She grows very serious and sometimes raises her voice as she expresses the full measure of her passion for nursing.

Celeste knows that some of her colleagues are annoyed when she does this. Their behaviors say it all: they stop making eye contact, they verbally cut her off, and they show other signs that they don't want to listen when she speaks.

Celeste is committed to being more successful at persuading others to come around to her point of view. She wants to know what she is doing to lose the interest and active support of her peers. What do you think? Why is it that Hannah can motivate her fellow health care professionals to participate in initiatives that go beyond what's required, and why is Celeste having trouble doing the same thing in a similar setting?

Why is passion "working" for Hannah but not for Celeste? Doesn't the literature tell us that when we tap into our passion, we tap into what truly motivates us? When we speak with heart-felt conviction, isn't that enough to inspire others who should be like-minded? When we reveal our sincerity and commitment, isn't that enough to convince those around us that our cause should be their cause too?

Simply stated, the answer is no. I hear from countless nurses that there are times when expressing the full measure of their enthusiasm for nursing just doesn't work. Despite the wisdom and direction their passion offers them, when they communicate it with zeal to others, sometimes it backfires and turns people off.

What is this about? And, if this has happened to you, what can you do about it? To answer this question, we need to take a look at these two leaders and see what they are doing differently. Let's start with Celeste, who is eager to understand why her communication strategy is not giving her the results she wants. She starts by drilling down and recalling the details of a recent situation in which her "audience" was turned off by her passion. The "audience" in this case was her boss. She could identify the exact moment in which he began to resist. She also remembered that her immediate, "unconscious" reaction to his opposition was to speak louder and add detail to emphasize the merits of her cause.

What is Hannah doing differently? She is just as excited as Celeste, but there is one significant difference in what she does in conversations in which she wants to persuade—even when such dialogue becomes contentious. It is this: Hannah is conscious of staying connected with the other person when they are speaking together. She conveys genuine interest in hearing their statements and positions. She is clear that showing this kind of attentiveness is central to achieving productive collaboration. She is equally clear that to hear others and to identify areas of common commitment helps achieve success rather than hinder it. Listening to others, even when they disagree, does not mean that she is abandoning her own position. Far from it, Hannah is interested in relating to the other person on his or her own terms *as well as* her own.

In other words, instead of experiencing concern or resistance as a threat that "requires" her to get more vocal about her own passion, Hannah seeks to understand the other person's priorities. She has learned that instead of getting more excited, she is more successful when she calms down. By taking this approach, through her attention and her actions, she is demonstrating that she is not just focused on herself but also equally focused on those with whom she is speaking, and she works to discover common ground so they can both win.

Behaving in ways that lead to mutual goal achievement sends a distinctly different message than repeatedly emphasizing only our own positions. Hannah is effective because she stays engaged with her audience rather than subtly but surely sending the message that she cares only about her own point of view.

Hannah also attends to several other aspects of her communication. She:

1. *Listens to herself and considers whether she is communicating clearly.*
2. *Thinks about whether her message is tailored to the current situation or whether she is sending the same message she always sends.* She knows that if her message does not vary, her predictable response can easily be discounted by her colleagues.

Hannah is effective because she stays in touch with others and what's happening in the present, in addition to tapping into her passion and how she articulates it. She knows that the most effective strategy is to stay connected with herself AND those around her.

Together, and only together, can they achieve what they all most want—to provide a better system of care for all their patients and communities.

20

The Art of the Question

When you are challenged by others, what do you do? Do you become curious and ask questions, and if so, what kinds of questions do you pose? Are they courteous invitations and requests to say more? Or are they "missiles"?[a] Do your queries open up dialogue or do they discourage inquiry and mutual exploration? Read on for ways your questions can lead to better communication, shared understanding, and workable ways forward.

Carmen was a competent department director who was frustrated with Megan, one of her nurse managers. She was concerned about Megan's difficulty with some of her management responsibilities, but her attempts to discuss these problems with Megan weren't working. Most recently, Megan was late with the performance reviews for her staff. Carmen asked Megan why she was late with the reviews, and Megan looked dumbfounded—almost as if Carmen's question was falling on deaf ears. So Carmen asked the question again, this time adding more volume and urgency. Again, Megan didn't answer. Carmen gave up, returned to her office, and grew increasingly frustrated.

Her irritation mounted as she thought about the other recent times when Megan "stonewalled" her questions or didn't perform as required, or both. She knew she couldn't keep asking Megan questions, since she just got blank stares in response. Therefore, she thought about putting Megan on a performance plan and, if necessary, making a personnel change. Finally, she concluded that she could not do that yet because there was too much going on in the organization, so she decided to just live with it.

Unfortunately, Carmen's thoughts about Megan and her decision to "live with it" came at a cost. But that cost was outside of her awareness: it was that her decision spawned even more resentment about Megan. Had Carmen been conscious of this, she probably would have said that

her increased anger was caused by Megan's actions. But Carmen's amplified bitterness did not come from anything Megan did or didn't do; it came from her own thoughts and decisions.

Rightly or wrongly, Carmen had concluded that she could not ask any more questions or put Megan on a performance plan. Although the latter choice might have been logical for Carmen, the former conclusion was not. She had not considered her questions or the way she was asking them, nor had she thought about whether her own behavior was escalating the issue.

Carmen also didn't realize that she had made a deal with herself when she decided to just live with it. That "deal" had many consequences, such as:

- Carmen would grow more, not less, frustrated with Megan's behavior.
- Carmen would probably not change the tone or the direction of her dialogue with Megan.
- Megan's behavior was unlikely to change.
- Megan's poor performance would affect others around her.
- Carmen's team and the organization would consequently suffer.

If we step away from the specifics, we can see that there are several ways in which Carmen can reverse these consequences. She has two options that are relatively easy and readily available. At least temporarily, she can shift the focus to herself and her own behavior, and shift her attention away from Megan. She can also change the quality of her questions and the tone she uses when asking them.

Turning her attention inward can increase Carmen's awareness of her own internal dialogue and the power she is giving to it. For example, she can reexamine her belief that she can't ask any more questions and she just has to live with it. Rather than dismissing the prospect of any more questions, she can rethink the ones she is asking and the way she is asking them. She can also consider her goals: What did she want to accomplish with her questions for Megan? What impact did she want to have on Megan?

---

[a]Adams M. *Guidelines for Great Question Askers*. Lambertville, NJ. The Inquiry Institute; 2011.

Was she simply asking for information? Or is it possible that Carmen also wanted to "make" Megan feel guilty and let her know that she was frustrated and angry? Although no leader wants to admit less-than-admirable motives, it is important to be honest with ourselves when we reflect on our own actions and intentions.

Marilee Adams offers a relevant perspective: "A question can be an invitation, a request, or a missile. What impact do you want your questions to have?" We don't know the history of Carmen's relationship with Megan, and we can't speculate on what impact Carmen wants to have now. However, we can look at her behavior and her words. Any question that starts with "why" can easily elicit a defensive response. Better choices for honest responses are words like how, what, and when. While questions that begin with these words can't guarantee positive results, they are far less likely to produce reactive, self-justifying answers.

Carmen can also change the tone she uses when she asks her questions. Although this seems easy enough, adjusting her tone will be more effective if she also changes her attitude. It is highly likely that Megan senses Carmen's irritation, and as a result, she may feel threatened or shamed, or both. Whatever Megan's feelings are, they are probably negative and undoubtedly contributing to her inability to respond.

If Carmen wants a different dialogue with Megan, her best option is to ask herself if she can have a positive attitude and listen to what Megan has to say. Perhaps Carmen can shift her stance from anger to curiosity. These internal changes may require real effort on Carmen's part, especially if she has been frustrated for any length of time. There are several ways by which she can increase the likelihood of being successful with her efforts to change her attitude:

1. *She can focus on whatever is constructive about Megan's work history or their past personal relationship.* If she can do this, it is likely that she can find more capacity to be positive and to question Megan accordingly. If she shifts her attitude, she is in a better position to ask questions that are not laden with a negative edge.

2. *If Carmen is too angry to become genuinely curious, she can try suspending her anger just for a short time.* She can tell herself that it will still be there when and if she wants it back. Meanwhile, she can try being open to a positive outcome and genuine curiosity. Even in difficult circumstances, most of us can momentarily let go of negative judgments and difficult feelings if we know we can return to them. When we do let go, even for a few moments, our attitudes and the quality of our questions can change dramatically. It's still possible that we won't get answers that are satisfactory, and it's also possible that people listening to our newfound positivity won't immediately accept and believe it. But if we keep it up and we still don't create better dialogue and good outcomes, at least we will have adjusted our own attitudes and become more skilled communicators.

Carmen wanted to experiment with these strategies. Although she was uncertain about whether she could develop a better rapport with Megan, she was willing to try. She was surprised and delighted when they were able to have several qualitatively different conversations. It wasn't long before she learned that Megan had significant family issues and minor, but disruptive, health concerns. Megan was embarrassed to tell Carmen about these problems, but she knew they were getting in the way of her job performance. Together, Carmen and Megan built a plan to help Megan get back on track. Carmen was especially happy because she had taken steps to improve her working relationships by increasing the effectiveness of her questions and examining her own behavior.

21

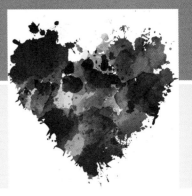

Coaching Up

Do you know how to coach your boss? "Coaching" your boss is not about subtle manipulation to get what you want. Instead, it is about effective communication that increases the chances of getting what you need by finding a common ground. It is also about being curious, respectful, and assertive so that your boss can better understand you and become a genuine collaborator and supporter.

A lot of nurse managers and leaders ask me how they can have better relationships with their bosses. The question comes in different forms, but the essence remains the same. See if you identify with any of these examples:

- "I need resources to get the job done, but whenever I approach my boss, she is preoccupied, doesn't listen, or just says 'no'."
- "My boss means well, but he doesn't understand what's going on in my unit."
- "I do a good job, and I feel like I've 'tried everything' to please my boss. Still, she seems to have made up her mind about my work, and her conclusion is negative."
- "I am doing well in my position. My boss encourages and believes in me. I have the potential to do a lot more, and I'd like my boss to mentor me, but she is so busy that I hesitate to ask."
- "My boss micromanages me."
- "I don't like my boss' values. All she thinks about is managing to the bottom line."
- "Despite my best efforts, I can't seem to communicate successfully with my boss (or the board or the CEO)."

These and other variations on the theme of strengthening our relationships with our bosses come up again and again in my executive coaching sessions. One best practice for managing this significant challenge is what I call "coaching up."

Just what is coaching up? Let's start with what it is not. It is not a calculating way to get the boss to see it our way. It is not borne of the belief that there is one right way—ours! Nor does it support a conscious or unconscious belief that the boss is wrong.

"Coaching up" means learning and using well-tested coaching and communication skills, which promote authentic, positive, and productive relationships with *all* of the individuals who are involved in our success. When coaching up techniques are applied to our most significant professional relationship, the boss, they enrich mutual understanding and often reduce frustration and stress.

While no specific tool ever guarantees success, coaching up techniques have a very good track record. Here are some examples of strategies for leaders:

GET INTO THE RIGHT FRAME OF MIND

When we are committed to coaching up, we work hard to suspend negative judgments about the boss, whether these are conscious and crystal clear or faint and subtle. Either way, these attitudes influence how we interact with our boss. Suspending them does not mean we have to delete them completely and forever, but it does mean that we need to put them aside at least temporarily. We need to do this so that they don't interfere with being fully present in our interactions. Focusing on the here and now means we engage from a position of genuine interest in improving our relationship with our boss.

BECOME CURIOUS

When we coach up, we move into a state of being that is genuinely curious and interested in our boss' point of view. We may want to know more about her position, how she feels about something, or what he needs to fully support us. These are just three examples of ways in which we can demonstrate our interest. There are many others.

LISTEN WITH RESPECT

From a place of openness, we listen with our full attention. We ask clarifying questions when needed, and we continue to disregard judgments and distractions that arise during our conversation. When we disagree, we try to become even more curious. We ask questions like "What factors are influencing this decision?" or "Please help me understand this."

PRACTICE THE ART OF THE QUESTION

We ask open-ended questions rather than questions that are answered with "yes" or "no." To invite dialogue, we begin our questions with "how" and "what" as often as we can.

MANAGE PARADOX

While effective leaders know their options and plans, they are also open to shifting gears if they receive persuasive new information. They know that they may not always have the full picture of what's involved in the complex challenge of running a health care organization. This is particularly true when working with bosses who have a much broader organizational perspective than we do.

COMMUNICATE REQUESTS AND NEEDS CLEARLY

In my coaching, I often encounter nurse leaders and managers who are passionate and clear about their solutions. However, when we role-play or discuss how they communicate with their bosses, their commitments can come out sounding wishy-washy, diluted, or filled with qualifiers that would confuse any listener. Sometimes this happens because the leader does not articulate clearly. But often it's because mental chatter is preventing her from speaking effectively.

ATTEND TO YOUR BOSS'S COMMUNICATION AND LEARNING STYLE

Some learners are visual, while others are auditory. Some like big picture information, while others prefer lots of detail; some like crisp bullet points, others like longer pieces; some like to be told after actions have been taken, and some like to know our every step before and during our tasks. Do you know your boss' communication preferences? If not, it's time for a curious conversation!

NEGOTIATE YOUR DIFFERENCES

For example, if your boss likes to be informed of your unit's key activities on a daily basis, ask how she would like to receive that information. If she says she wants a written report, and you don't have the time to compose that each day, ask if she would accept a weekly written report, along with a daily phone message covering the day's highlights. She may say yes, and she may say no. If she says no, offer another solution that will meet her needs as well as your own.

UNDERSTAND VALUES' DIFFERENCES AND SEEK TO FIND COMMON GROUND

You may not agree with your boss' values (e.g., being driven by the bottom line vs. providing high-quality patient care), but there may be ways to coexist. From a position of inquisitiveness, discover what is important to your boss. For instance, at an appropriate time, ask what prompted her to go into health care or what she most likes about her work. Chances are she will divulge something that you can appreciate or understand. This can create a sense of common ground and shared values, at least to some extent. Knowing and valuing your boss' history may give you something in common on which to build. As you continue to coach up, you may improve your opinion and feelings about your boss.

SHARE YOUR PERSPECTIVE AND OPENLY ASK FOR YOUR BOSS'S POINT OF VIEW

When you are discussing an important mutual concern, ask questions like, "What are you seeing that I am not seeing?" If your boss wants your help with something, ask, "How can I support you?" If you want your boss's backing or mentoring, be specific about the ways you want your boss to support you. Ask what you can do to make it possible for her to say yes.

These and similar strategies are what I call coaching up. When we use this approach, we are taking the initiative to form a respectful and supportive relationship with the boss. We are laying the groundwork for a positive and productive alliance, and we are significantly enhancing our chances of successfully working together.

Even if negative judgments do creep back in from time to time, we have tools to work toward mutual understanding, if we choose to use them. Coaching up isn't a magic bullet, but it is a very good way to enrich your partnership with your boss—that most significant of all organizational relationships.

22

Listen and Speak with Care

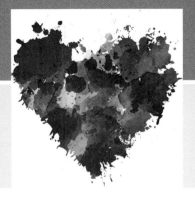

Many experts say that leadership is all about communication. If that's true, how are we talking about our work and our challenges? Are we speaking truthfully and with care? Or are our narratives biased, discouraging, and pessimistic? How can we communicate more thoughtfully and positively with others and with ourselves?

Many of us think about listening as a leadership competency that, when done well, requires the full measure of our presence. Our experience tells us that attentive, skillful listening rewards us with better relationships and improved outcomes. Although these beliefs are true enough, they rest on the assumption that listening is primarily about hearing other people. Although that is accurate as far as it goes, a different kind of listening is at least as important, that is, listening to ourselves.

Recently an established and close group of health care and nurse leaders from across the country spent a few days together. As part of their work, they shared tales of their successes and stories about their challenges. When it was time to drill down on their challenges, more than a few of their accounts were layered with a good degree of emotional angst.

The participants felt safe together, and they offered empathy and support to one another as they listened to the commentaries. Here are a few examples offered in detail-free form: "I have to do this, and it will never work" and "I've got to do that, and I have never succeeded in doing anything like it before." There were also statements like "This is just the way I am" and "(Someone else) is stopping me from being successful."

They exchanged heartfelt offers of mutual assistance, and the atmosphere of "we're in this together" was palpable. Yet, the group's collective body language demonstrated an altogether different reality. Some participants looked a bit hunched, and the rest exuded more than a hint of loss. They were not sitting tall. Indeed, they were far from the excited leaders they had been moments before, when they

had spoken about the highlights of their many accomplishments. There was a heavy sense of defeat in the air.

These leaders demonstrated what happens when the press of too much to do limits our capacities to consider how we think about and describe our own experiences. Although the members of the group paid rapt attention to one another as they spoke, they appeared to be less conscious of truly listening to what they themselves were saying. Even if they were attentive to their own words, they seemed to be unaware of the negative impact of those words—not just on other people but also on themselves.

They also seemed to miss the limits of what they were saying. Most spoke as if there were only one perspective available to them. For understandable reasons, they probably had allocated little time to reflect and, consequently, they had generated that single "truth." That became *the* truth they believed and subsequently shared with those around them.

What if these leaders could listen as attentively to what they were saying to themselves as they did to the others? While honoring their feelings and standpoints, could they also imagine new, *equally valid* ways of looking at their experiences? If so, what potential could those equally valid viewpoints offer? What might these different perspectives release in these leaders and, eventually, in the people around them?

Those in attendance were very interested in exploring diverse and more effective ways of leaning into, yet getting beyond, their current perspectives and feelings. They were especially concerned with moving forward to meet their challenges powerfully and with the full measure of their leadership abilities.

Here is what they did to shift their downbeat narratives:

1. **They literally "set aside" the original yet adverse version of the truth that they had shared with the group.** They knew they could reclaim every word and nuance any time they wanted. In the meantime, however, each of them agreed to simply let those first versions go for a while so they could explore alternative ways of listening to and thinking about themselves.

2. ***They repeated their stories, but not in their original form.*** This time, they added more to them. For example, "I want to change my approach, but I can't" grew to include what that belief allowed for. So, "I want to change my approach, but I can't" expanded to include "…and so I will 'skill up.' I will better equip myself by taking classes in communication effectiveness and assertiveness training."

3. ***They said what they will do the next time they have this challenge.*** Thus, "I want to change my approach, but I can't" became "and although I have believed that I can't, the next time I feel this way, I will practice a different approach. For example, I will be more assertive, and I will ask for what I need. I know I may feel uncomfortable doing this initially, but eventually, I will get good at it."

4. ***They conceptually agreed that events have many potential interpretations, and that there is more than one equally valid point of view.*** This shift opened up new possibilities for each of them. They experimented with different ways of describing what they were facing by answering questions like "what else could you say about this?"

5. ***After articulating alternative, truthful, and eventually more positive ways of framing their challenges, they selected the one that was most authentic and affirming.*** They said out loud "…and the most positive yet honest way I can look at this is…." As they did this, these leaders' energies shifted dramatically. There was also a lot of laughter in the room.

6. ***They talked about what they really wanted to accomplish going forward.*** This allowed them to anchor their challenges, feelings, and their self-talk in their individual, positive, and authentic aspirations instead of their negative beliefs.

When these leaders concluded these exercises, not a single person opted to go back to his or her original story. Their physical and emotional affects were quite different than earlier in the day. They achieved these results by tuning in and listening to themselves. Each honored his original story, but no one stuck to it "no matter what." They demonstrated what is possible if we as leaders listen more carefully to ourselves and truly attend to the renditions of fact that we tell ourselves and others.

23

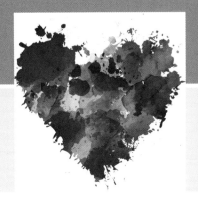

Leadership and Betrayal

You feel you have been betrayed at work. Betrayal takes many forms, and experts say that it happens to 90% of us. What can we do to understand and handle on-the-job betrayals? What can we do to move beyond our disappointment and engage in constructive action?

As an executive coach, I am frequently told about nurses' experiences at the helm. Sometimes these are inspired tales of persistence and triumph, often in the face of profound adversity.

But sometimes these leaders' stories reveal vulnerability, deep wounds, and major defeats. Although a single word can't do justice to their feelings, a few reflect their spirit: disappointment, duplicity, disloyalty, and even heartbreak.

I do not offer these descriptions lightly. Look around you. Look within yourself. It is highly likely that you and I and most of us have faced at least one betrayal at work. In fact, trust experts Drs. Dennis and Michelle Reina report that betrayal is universal and that 90% of employees experience betrayal frequently in the workplace.[a]

THE MANY FORMS OF BETRAYAL

According to Merriam-Webster, to "betray" means to be led astray, to deliver to an enemy, and to fail or desert, especially in times of need.[b] In nursing leadership, betrayal can take many forms, including situations like these:

[a]Reina D, Reina M. *Rebuilding Trust in the Workplace.* San Francisco, CA: Berrett-Koehler; 2010.
[b]Betray. Merriam-Webster website. http://www.Merriam-Webster .com.

"After years of nurturing solid relationships with my peers and superiors, my boss told me that I will be reporting to someone I do not respect. I was not asked for my opinion before this change was broadly announced."
- "As a leader nearing the end of my career, I agreed to put my life's work in another's hands. I believed what I was told—that the work I constructed would continue. I have since learned that my work has been changed so radically that it no longer resembles what I created."
- "Without giving me a chance to advise my staff, my boss went around me and contacted my team members to seek opinions about my leadership."
- "No matter how much I listen, or how hard I try to understand and deliver what is expected, I cannot seem to provide my supervisor what she needs. I feel that I am being forced to leave."

OUR MANY RESPONSES TO BETRAYAL

Our responses can take many forms too:
- Sometimes a leader dons a mask and creates a well-honed story that allows him to save face as he appears to move on. But when that same leader has a chance, he shares stories and feelings that tell a different story. We discover that he has not processed or come to terms with what occurred. Instead, he harbors bitterness and resentment.
- Some leaders are indignant. "How could this have happened to me? I've always had excellent performance evaluations, I have had a lot of feedback about the quality of my leadership, and I have led my part of this organization in very challenging circumstances. I have done everything I could. I simply don't understand."

- Some leaders form a sub-rosa plan to achieve fairness and reciprocity. Said another way, they launch a thinly disguised effort to get even.
- Some leaders believe that their most important professional relationships are no longer trustworthy. Consequently, they question their own judgment, the other party's character, or both.
- Some leaders question their competence. They thought they were good leaders, perhaps even great leaders. They have lots of evidence to prove it, but their confidence is deeply shaken. They wonder what happened. How could they have made such a significant miscalculation?

Merriam-Webster says that trust is the assured reliance on character, strength, ability, or the truth of someone or something. We place our confidence in those we trust.[c] Notice that in each of the earlier examples, there is a universal theme—trust has been broken.

So, what are we to make of broken trust and betrayal? If we consider our own experiences, we may ask many questions. If we stay long enough, are we bound to be betrayed? Is broken trust inevitable? Is it a consequence of being part of a diverse workforce that doesn't always share our values? Does betrayal increase in stressful times? Is it human nature to embrace the status quo and to feel betrayed when circumstances change?

HANDLING A BETRAYAL

If betrayal is so ubiquitous, what must we do when it occurs?

1. *We can consider whether the betrayal was intentional.* Drs. Denis and Michelle Reina have found that "90%

to 95% of the betrayals that cause problems at work are just the little ways we let people down."[d]

2. *We can consider the magnitude of the betrayal, acknowledge our emotions, and clarify what the betrayal really was.* We can also thoughtfully identify the betrayer. Was it our boss, coworker, or someone else? Or was it truly impersonal? Was it a position that the organization took that upset us?

3. *When betrayal happens at the hand of other people, we can ask ourselves whether we contributed to it.* Did we unwittingly aid and abet the betrayer? Maybe we didn't do our due diligence before making an agreement. Perhaps our emotions got ahead of the evidence, and we ignored signs that a betrayal was coming. Perhaps we were distracted. Perhaps we didn't attend to those whose legitimate organizational needs were not being met.

4. *Was the betrayal something that happened within us?* Did we abandon our own intentions and values? Were we not clear about what we needed, wanted, or believed? Were we silent when we should have spoken?

After having acknowledged our own feelings and having learned from the experience, we are more prepared to move on. Moving on can include forgiving others and being merciful with ourselves.

If a betrayal happened to us, we can offer ourselves the gift of reflection, grieving the loss and gaining wisdom from the experience. Yes, it can be very tempting to react, bury the pain, and move on, but if we do this, we miss the opportunity to learn and truly heal.

---

[c]Trust. Merriam-Webster website. http://www.Merriam-Webster.com.

[d]Wegel J. Rebuilding trust at work. *Chicago Tribune.* April 22, 2011. Available at: http://articles.chicagotribune.com/

24

Recognizing Competing Commitments

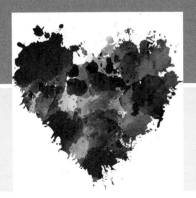

We believe our colleagues have failed us and we think we know the meaning of their disappointing behavior. When this happens, can we be curious and seek to understand before we condemn? Can we be open to discovering what is going on with our coworkers rather than making assumptions about what their actions mean?

Sally complained about her boss' behavior. Sally is the director of a service line in a large metropolitan hospital. She wrote to say that her boss, Linda, is wavering about a new program to which she had committed a few months earlier. The program is strategically important because it authorizes a new nursing role designed to improve the quality of patient outcomes and satisfaction. Based on Linda's earlier commitment to the initiative, Sally interviewed several nurses who were enthusiastic about the new positions. Sally also generated excitement among her existing nursing staff.

Now, it appears that Linda, the chief operating officer, is backpedaling on her earlier promise. Sally does not understand why Linda changed her mind, and she is angry and disappointed.

Nora, another reader, writes about her frustration with "the lack of integrity" of one of her direct reports. Nora says that she has repeatedly asked Henry, a nurse manager, to turn in performance evaluations for his nurses. Henry promises to turn in the evaluations, but on three separate occasions he has not done so.

What do these scenarios have in common? Both Linda and Henry are not following through on what they said they were going to do. Sally and Nora are understandably upset by behaviors they view as irresponsible and unacceptable. What should they do now? Should Sally act on her disappointment in her boss' recent behavior? She says she wants to leave her position and work at the hospital across town.

Nora is clear that integrity is a very important value to her, and she is equally clear that she does not want a nurse manager who has "no integrity" reporting to her. Nora says she is ready to go to HR to initiate the process of firing Henry.

Here is the important point: our readers are ready to act based on the information they have and what they believe it means. *But both Nora and Sally are interpreting the actions of their colleagues in only one way.*

Are there are any other ways to explain Linda and Henry's behavior?

Obviously, something is stopping Henry and Linda from honoring their earlier commitments. Both are well-regarded nurses, so it is unlikely they have suddenly become wishy-washy and untrustworthy. Yet, notice that neither Nora nor Sally has asked what is preventing their colleagues from moving forward with the commitments they made. Interestingly, neither has offered support by asking how she might help.

If Sally and Nora were to engage differently, they might be able to learn about Henry and Linda's current concerns or aspirations. In other words, they might be able to hear about the pressing commitments that are *more important* to Linda and Henry *right now*.

In their seminal Harvard Business Review article "The Real Reason People Won't Change,"[a] Kegan and Lahey describe the very real impact of multiple and sometimes competing commitments on human behavior. Health care leaders, for example, may be committed to improving the quality of patient care through all available means. Simultaneously, however, they are also committed to holding down costs. They know that if there is "no margin," there is "no mission."

Sometimes leaders may be dealing with more subtle competing commitments. For example, an otherwise exemplary employee may come late to work or miss it altogether because of challenges with a spouse or child. Although the hospital worker is still strongly committed

[a]Kegan R, Lahey L. The real reason people won't change. *Harvard Business Review*. 2001;79(11):85–92.

to satisfactory job performance, he is attending to his personal needs and unable to negotiate a solution that will allow him to continue to perform well.

These examples illustrate the importance of learning more about what is causing otherwise good managers to perform in unexpected ways. As leaders, we must practice the art of discovery. This means having the ability to create a conversation that allows additional information to come forward.

Do we need to become employee assistance program officers, therapists, or detectives? No! Here are several proven strategies:

Suspend unhelpful assumptions and judgments. When we can set aside our own biases and premature conclusions, we can listen openly. When we authentically listen, we encourage dialogue that is both real and trusting. We are in a better position to elicit the truth.

Become curious. Would it be possible for Nora to temporarily suspend her belief that Henry lacks integrity? If yes, she could become genuinely curious about what is preventing Henry from turning in his performance evaluations.

Listen for what is not being said. Listen to more than words. What is the emotional tone of the person with whom you are concerned? What do you read in her body language? What might be in their way?

Manage internal barriers that interfere with listening and communicating. When we are listening, are we preparing what we are going to say next or are we genuinely hearing the other person? Are we listening generously and to understand? Are we summarizing what we are hearing so the other person knows she is being heard?

Nora and Sally decided to use these techniques in ways that were comfortable and natural for them. Sally chose to speak with her boss Linda about her apparent change of heart. Sally was careful to practice the conversation before the meeting to avoid becoming angry with Linda. This preparation served her well. She was able to have an honest dialogue in which Linda indicated that supporting this expensive program was no longer a position she could take with the CEO and executive committee of the hospital. Without embarrassing Linda, Sally surmised that Linda was afraid to take what she perceived as a big risk.

With this new information, Sally was able to offer support to Linda. She proposed to accompany Linda to the next executive team meeting to provide data and explain the projected outcomes of the new program. In other words, Sally was willing to take on some of the risk that Linda was experiencing.

It does not matter whether we agree that Linda *should* feel this way or that Sally is willing to take on risk for her boss. What matters is that our reader demonstrated a willingness to listen for her boss' deeper commitment. Because she heard Linda's aversion to taking this risk with the executive team, she was able to propose a solution and move the project forward.

Our other reader, Nora, temporarily suspended her judgment about Henry's lack of integrity. She engaged him using the tools above, and what she learned completely surprised her. Henry had been trained in the military, and he was embarrassed to let Nora know that he did not know how to conduct the performance evaluations.

We may have opinions about how and whether this could have happened, but we can learn from this reader's real experience. Although Henry was committed to excellence in nursing management, *in this case, he was more committed to saving face with his boss.* Nora could never have discovered this had she not created enough safety and comfort for their conversation.

25

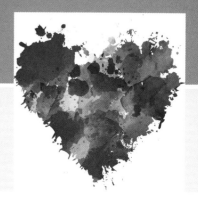

Your Evaluation Doesn't Go Well. What Will You Do?

Your performance review didn't go well and you're upset about the feedback you've received from your boss. How can you discard what's unimportant yet stay open to understanding and accepting what is important from your boss's perspective? What can you do to hear what was said while maintaining your emotional equanimity, sense of self-worth, and personal power?

In my work, I encounter many questions about handling difficult challenges with bosses. The queries come in equal measure from leaders and managers. They come from all levels and many organizational settings. This is not surprising, since nothing is more important to many leaders than having a good or at least a productive and respectful relationship with their supervisors.

In January 2005, the Harvard Business Review reprinted a time-honored article from 1973 entitled "Managing Your Boss,"[a] citing its still potent message in 2005. Based on my anecdotal experience, I believe the topic is just as universal and relevant today. This column is about a leader's experience with her evaluation and how the relationship with her boss went astray. It also focuses on what the leader did to fix it. Although this tale is about a particular circumstance, its teachings apply to many interactions between our bosses and ourselves.

Anna is a nurse leader who has held her position for 5 years. She has been widely acknowledged for the outcomes she has achieved since taking over an already successful operation. She has introduced improvements on existing services, implemented new services in accordance with the overall strategic plan, and improved her operation's metrics on nearly every dimension.

Anna has enjoyed positive working relationships with her peers and other leaders with whom she regularly interacts, and her relationships with her immediate bosses were positive as well. In the 5 years that she has been in the position, she has had three supervisors. Eleanor, her most recent supervisor, arrived 2 years ago.

Anna's yearly evaluation was due 6 months after Eleanor started. Much to Anna's surprise, both the data collection process and outcome were different from what she expected. The previous process of gathering and delivering feedback from various sources was changed without her prior knowledge. When she learned of the changes, it was too late for her to ask for adjustments.

One of Anna's concerns was that the endpoint for the data-gathering period was ill defined. Her concern was justified: Anna's review was scheduled with little notice and poor choices of times and venues. Thus, the meeting took place at an inconvenient hour and location. She and Eleanor did not have sufficient time to review the results together, and their meeting did not occur in a comfortable or private setting.

The evaluation results were much less positive than Anna expected; to make matters worse, the ways in which she could improve were unclear. Anna was both frustrated and angry. Most of all, she was disappointed with the process and the lack of clarity on how to be successful.

But she did not seek more information or a better understanding of what Eleanor and others wanted. So, for the next year, Anna attempted to lead her organization in ways that she assumed would be satisfactory to those evaluating her. There was no structured or unstructured "check in" with her boss to determine how she was doing. Nine months into the year, when Anna's next evaluation was 3 months away, she made requests for adjustments in the coming evaluation process. A few of her requests were granted, others were not. Although the resulting evaluation procedure was more acceptable to her than last time, the results were even more negative than before. The only consolation was that the expectations were much clearer than they had been previously.

[a]Gabarro J, Kotter J. Managing your boss. *Harv Bus Rev*. January, 2005. http://hbr.org/2005/01/managing-your-boss/ar/1. Accessed August 29, 2012.

To say that Anna was distraught after receiving the second evaluation is an understatement. Still, she soldiered on while harboring many uncomfortable and unproductive feelings. After 6 months, she decided to seek executive coaching.

WHAT WOULD YOU DO IN THIS SITUATION?

Here's what happened with Anna. First, to be a successful leader again, she had to acknowledge her feelings about these evaluations. She quickly uncovered the layers of emotions that had engulfed her for 18 months. She blamed Eleanor for changing the "rules" of her evaluation without informing or involving her. She also blamed Eleanor for surprising her with an unsatisfactory evaluation and not being specific about what Anna needed to do to be effective going forward.

Anna also realized that she had let these feelings fester while she tried to address unclear expectations. She grieved the results of the second evaluation, and she also reflected on how surprising they were, particularly because she felt she had done so much to improve.

All of Anna's reactions are understandable and human. However, they still took a heavy toll on her emotionally and physically. They also rendered her unable to assertively handle the challenges before her.

So, what are the remedies in a situation like this? Here's what Anna says she would do differently now. Her solutions fall into the following two categories.

ACT SOONER

There are many junctures at which Anna sees that she did not stand up for herself. She failed to take action, and she failed to take it in a timely way. Some of those instances are:

- Her acceptance of unclear expectations in the first evaluation with Eleanor
- Her decision to move forward for 12 months on the basis of assumptions about what Eleanor and others wanted versus a clear understanding of what they wanted
- Her willingness to live in ambiguity and discomfort despite the importance of her work to patients and the importance of Eleanor's satisfaction with her performance
- Her frustration with the change in evaluation process but her decision to wait 9 months to address it
- Her failure to deal with her pent-up feelings of disrespect and disregard as a professional
- Her allowance of a 12-month lapse between meetings in which she would receive feedback

FACE CRITICISM AND HANDLE IT WITH CARE

Anna realized that her lack of proactivity was a result of her inability to take in the negative feedback. Like many leaders, it was emotionally challenging for Anna to hear that she was not doing well when she was used to being successful. She knows that she should not take it personally, but despite what she knows intellectually, she *does* take it personally.

What she says she would do now is solicit feedback more frequently and make sure she understands it. Rather than holding on to being emotionally hurt by the input, she would ask herself if she agrees with it. Even if the whole feedback does not register as true, she would consider whether there might be some part of it that is.

Anna's incentive to act differently is powerful; she has tried the alternative and the results were quite painful. Accepting and acting on ambiguous expectations did not work. She is acutely aware that her efforts for 12 months not only missed the mark but also fostered an even more negative review.

Anna has reflected a lot on what happened, and she has compassion for herself and her mistakes. But she is also clear about what she has learned. As she unburdened herself, she became more able to speak up and act on her own behalf. Consequently, Anna directly approached Eleanor and asked for a meeting to review how she was doing well in advance of her next evaluation. Eleanor was agreeable and, at Anna's request, before the meeting, Eleanor sought feedback from the others who would formally provide it in a few months.

During their meeting, Eleanor spoke for the group. She provided a positive feedback about many of Anna's efforts. She also said there were areas in which Anna was not yet producing the results that she and others wanted to see.

Anna considered these assessments, and they all made sense to her. She put remedies in place for the problem areas, and when her formal evaluation occurred a few months later, the results were quite positive. Perhaps just as significant, Anna felt much better about herself and her willingness to learn and grow.

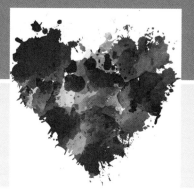

26

The Downside of Storytelling

One of your direct reports is not performing as you think he should. You assume you understand his problem, and as time passes, you become more convinced of your story, even though it is wrong. Can you step back from your certainty and discover how you are contributing to this escalating challenge?

This is a tale about Amy, a busy leader with a vexing challenge. For 11 months, Amy had been the director of an emergency room in a large urban hospital. She is a seasoned, skilled nurse leader who is well intentioned and inspired to do her best.

Recently, she became very frustrated with one of her direct reports, William. During most of her tenure on this job, Amy found William to be a competent nurse manager. But lately, she experienced him as evasive and even secretive about a key facet of his role—providing timely, written feedback to his direct reports and completing the organization's performance review documentation. Amy knows that many nurse managers do not like this aspect of their positions, but most understand the importance of the task and do it anyway.

Amy was convinced there was something amiss with William. She described their interactions with palpable exasperation. She asked him for his written reviews several times, but each time he offered a different excuse and a new date by which she would have them. Each time, he did not come through, and Amy grew more upset. Each time, she went back and restated her need for those evaluations.

The next time, William looked away and dodged the question when Amy approached him yet again. Amy believed William's response demonstrated "willful" disregard for her wishes. This ratcheted up her emotions and angered her even more. Although she had been reluctant to start him on a performance plan, she was now convinced that it was her only choice. She said she was mentally prepared to move him out of his role altogether.

If we step back from the details, we see that Amy continued to do the same things with William over and over

again. When he did not comply, also over and over, she became emotionally overwrought and increasingly engaged with her own story about what he was doing: stubbornly disregarding her wishes. By the time she discussed this with me, she was determined to levy serious consequences for his "insubordination."

TELLING VS ASKING

Stepping even farther back, we can see that Amy is completely wrapped up in her own emotions, her need for resolution, and her interpretation of William's actions. When we talked, Amy recognized that she had never asked him what was preventing him from turning in his evaluations. In hindsight, she wondered how she could have missed such an obvious question. Soon, she realized that she missed it because, like most leaders, she had many responsibilities, needed to move fast, and wanted to obtain results in the most direct way. All she could see was that he was not cooperating, and those performance reviews had to be completed. They were in fact, many, many months late!

Amy's emotions were coupled with her need for speed and her story about the meaning of William's actions. This potent combination narrowed her ability to think. In that state, she neglected to understand that no matter how many times she told him what to do, she was not going to be successful.

In her book *Change Your Questions Change Your Life*, Marilee G. Adams posits that a truly effective communication comprises 20% telling and 80% asking.[a] Amy and many of us have this ratio turned around. A profound change can occur in ourselves and those around us when we stop relying on our statements and start learning from our questions. When our leadership approaches are not working, we can expand our chances for success by opening our minds to the new wisdom that curiosity evokes.

[a]Adams MG. *Change Your Questions Change Your Life*. San Francisco, CA: Berrett-Koehler Publishers; 2004.

Through this simple yet significant shift, we can detach from our steadfast but perhaps erroneous interpretations of "the truth." In this case, Amy's conviction about the "truth" of William's behavior was contributing to her ineffective leadership. She also realized that when she described William's behavior as "insubordinate," she became even angrier and more resentful. If anyone had asked, she would have said that his behavior was generating those feelings. But upon reflection, she knew that what actually created those feelings was the emotionally charged story she told herself about his actions.

Once Amy grasped that she had never asked what was preventing William from completing the evaluations, she accepted that she contributed to the impasse with him. She was willing, at least temporarily, to suspend her belief that she was right about the meaning of his behavior and became genuinely curious.

What she learned astounded her. Although William had been in the organization for several years, he had missed the training for performance reviews. He was a proud young professional, and he was embarrassed that he did not know how to do this part of his job. He didn't know how to tell Amy that he was simply not competent in this way. Her continual reproaches made it very difficult for him to break through his own fear and shame.

It may be difficult to believe this simple story, but it is true. A nurse leader who is dedicated to doing her best and is acknowledged for her skill as a leader was about to dismiss an employee who was too proud to admit what he did not know. With her newfound knowledge, Amy supported William as he got the training he needed. He then ably fulfilled his responsibilities, and he and Amy began a new and more productive relationship.

What did Amy do to facilitate this turnaround?

1. *She was willing to entertain possible limitations in her judgment, and she released her attachment to being "right" about William's behavior.*
2. *She was willing to calm down and suspend, at least temporarily, her anger and frustration.*
3. *She realized that the problem she was experiencing was at least as much her responsibility as it was William's.* He was not performing as she needed him to perform, but she was not able to engage him in a way that allowed him to say what was preventing him from doing this part of his job.
4. *She set her intention:* she genuinely wanted to know the answers to the questions she asked William, and she genuinely wanted to listen.
5. *She began a new dialogue by letting William know that she wanted to talk openly with him.* She said she realized that her way of approaching him in recent conversations may not have been helpful.
6. *Her previous belief that William was a good nurse manager helped Amy shift her demeanor with him.* When she said, "I didn't handle this very well," her honesty sent a signal that helped William to be honest too. (She may well have chosen a different stance with a manager who was not an otherwise good performer.)
7. *Amy asked curious, open-ended questions.* She stayed away from leading questions and avoided the word "why" because she knew it could evoke defensiveness.

Amy's tale illustrates the power of releasing, even momentarily, our certainty and strong emotions when they may not be warranted. The behavioral portal for this powerful change is a simple shift from telling to asking. Amy's change of course shows us how the best leaders can let go of their stories and habits long enough to stop talking, start asking, and keep learning.

27

Leading a Team That's Checked Out

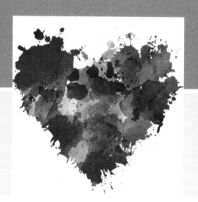

Your team is disengaged and you are frustrated. What can you do? First, realize that you are not alone. Many, if not most, workers in all fields are either not engaged or actively disengaged, according to the Gallup Organization.[a] But health care professionals can be different. Health care is a calling for many of us, including our staff, and there ARE workable strategies to reengage your team members so that they are more committed and productive.

At a recent gathering of nurse leaders, one of the participants, Callie, approached me with an obvious concern. She began by saying that her team is "checked out." She went on to describe her direct reports as a group of eight nurse leaders who are "waiting for retirement."

Callie also told that me she was recently promoted and she inherited this team. She is 10 to 15 years younger than her colleagues, and she believes they are only interested in doing what is minimally required to keep their jobs. She says that they do not contribute in meetings, and they are not willing to advance her vision-driven agenda for their department.

Is Callie the only nurse leader with a team of checked out members? Unfortunately, no! Although the settings and circumstances differ, there are numerous health care teams that operate with only partial engagement by their members.

In fact, in its 2017 *State of the Global Workplace* report,[a] the Gallup Organization found that in the 155 countries studied, only 15% of employees are engaged, or "highly involved in and enthusiastic" about work. In the United States and Canada, Gallup found that only 31%[b] are engaged. Gallup further explains that "engaged" employees are "psychologically committed to their jobs and likely to be making positive contributions to their organizations."

WHY AREN'T THEY ENGAGED?

So, Callie's team could be any team, and the reasons for their lack of engagement can vary greatly. Just a few could be disaffected team members who feel that they:
- "Don't like it here"
- "Don't like you as the manager"
- "Have too much to do, and you, the manager, don't get it"
- "Have too many priorities"
- "Are too busy to participate in these meetings, and you, the manager, are wasting my time"
- "Are better than/don't deserve this"

Notice that these attitudes are all forms of resistance that can translate into unproductive behavior such as undermining the manager's initiatives, not showing up for meetings, or not participating when they do attend.

But what about the manager? What can happen to Callie and any of us when we are in charge of a team with disengaged members? Here are some of the dynamics that can occur:

1. It can be tempting to "storytell" about these team members. *Storytelling* is what I call a *leadership seduction* in my book, *Leading Valiantly*,[c] and although Callie is a leader who excels, she has fallen prey to her own

---

[a]2017 State of the Global Workplace. GALLUP PRESS 1330 Avenue of the Americas 17th Floor New York, NY 10019 Library of Congress Control Number: 2017957145.

[b]Page 183 of the Gallup report referenced previously.
[c]Robinson-Walker C. *Leading Valiantly in Healthcare: Four Steps to Sustainable Success.* Indianapolis, IN: Sigma Theta Tau International. Honor Society of Nursing; 2013.

story about her team. Her story that they are waiting for retirement is strong enough to become a belief that stops her from imagining any other explanation for their behavior.

2. Even if she is correct, Callie's conviction has led her to conclude that nothing can be done except wait right along with them. Her belief is so strong that it blinds her to any other choice.

3. Team leaders like Callie can be so swept up in their stories that they forget the costs of inaction. Doing nothing about unproductive team members and whole teams with bad attitudes and poor performance can have real consequences, such as compromised patient care and a significant drop in productivity.

4. Managers who do not address subordinates' negative behaviors and attitudes may lose the respect of other subordinates, particularly those who are interested in doing their best. It can be a major disincentive to "go the extra mile" when managers do not levy consequences on those who do not meet performance standards or stated expectations.

5. Another consequence is that "actively disengaged" employees (19% in the United States and Canada) may be "actively engaged" in campaigns to enroll others in their pessimism. Employees who are particularly susceptible to signing up for negativity are those who fall into the "not engaged" category or 42% of all US and Canadian workers.

6. Finally, the manager herself may be tempted to check out too. Why? Because it's easier to look the other way, focus on other priorities, and choose "benign neglect." But when we too are tempted to resist and disengage, is the result really benign? What if there are consequences that affect patient care, directly or indirectly? What if there are other exceptional nurses who will notice that that the leader is not addressing the problem? What if Callie is regarded as a role model and mentor? What if there are goals that need active support from the team members who have not completely "left the building"? Will high-potential nurses feel it is fair to ask some team members to contribute while other team members have a free "pass"?

WHAT CAN YOU DO?

So, what can a manager do? Here are a few options that Callie can consider:

1. *She can monitor her own attitudes and stories.* Is it really true that every one of these eight individuals is not interested in offering anything more to the patients, team, and organization? Callie may have inadvertently closed herself off from other ways of seeing what's occurring. If she too has "checked out" of productively engaging with the team, her team members probably know it. If they do, they have even less reason to fully participate in the work of the department.

2. It is likely that Callie can't know whether any team members are capable of greater contribution without getting more information. One option she has is to *undertake team development.* On the front end, she or a trusted advisor can conduct a survey or set of interviews with the team.

3. *Callie can be transparent with the team* about why she is doing this, letting them know that she wants them to be professionally fulfilled, optimally productive, and that she wants to elicit their candid feedback about how things are going for them now. If she does this, she will need to assure the team that their responses will be anonymous.

4. *She could solicit their ideas for creating the environment in which greater productivity will occur,* and she can ask for the teams' thoughts about what is in the way of greater productivity now. Again, she will need to build trust and assure safety.

5. When she has the results, she and/or her advisor will want to *debrief the findings with the team.* This, too, is a process that should be undertaken with care. The team leader will want to state and respond to complaints realistically, be open and willing to change what can be changed, and be explicit about what cannot be changed.

These steps represent the beginning of team reengagement strategies, and they are just examples. Although they may not be appropriate for all teams, they do illustrate how leaders can address their own roles in team dysfunction and create the potential for greater engagement by everyone. When leaders shift their own attitudes and behaviors, it is more likely that at least some of the disengaged team members will change too.

28

Preparing Your Team for the Future

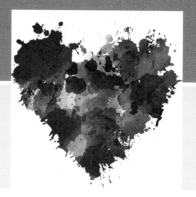

How ready is your team to tackle their problems and create a better future? Here are some approaches for assessing their readiness for crafting and enlivening a new and compelling vision, achievable goals, and long-term success.

If I were to ask you to rate your ability to *inspire a shared vision* with your team, what would you say?

In their seminal book, *The Leadership Challenge*, James Kouzes and Barry Posner tell us that inspiring a shared vision is one of the five critical competencies for leaders.[a] Their work is based on research involving thousands of people in all sectors, including health care. Yet when I ask nursing leaders and managers to rate their skills in this area, they invariably give themselves low scores. And in my coaching and consulting engagements, this same challenge presents itself again and again.

Readers of the Coaching Forum regularly ask about this too, so let's tackle it. While specific circumstances require individual attention that is beyond the reach of this column, some aspects of inspiring an engaging vision are universal. For example, there are ways to assess your group's *readiness* for an invigorated vision. Readiness is a key ingredient of success for any change initiative, and a revitalized vision may represent a significant change for your team. Addressing readiness increases your likelihood of eliciting a vision that is alive, fresh, and championed by others.

The following measures of readiness are culled from my practice and experience with many nurse leaders, as well as myriad other leadership and coaching experts. As you consider these questions, think about whether they apply to you. Please consider whether there are other indicators of readiness that are well suited for *your* team.

[a]Kouzes and Posner, *The Leadership Challenge: How to Make Extraordinary Things Happen in Organizations,* 6th Edition, Jossey-Bass; 6 edition. 2017, San Francisco, CA.

TEAM HISTORY

What significant organizational events have members of your team experienced recently? If there are newer members of the group, what have they heard about past events from the veterans? What are your team's beliefs about patient care and administration in your organization? How do the members of your team feel about the way nursing was managed in the past versus how it is being managed today? What stories and feelings do they have about you? Most important, how do these stories and beliefs affect your efforts to inspire a shared vision?

TEAM PERFORMANCE

How is the team performing? Are there factors that are propelling or undermining the group's effectiveness? If so, what are they? How can you address these issues so the team is ready to create an engaging, achievable, and sustainable vision?

TEAM VALUES

What core values do individuals on your team hold? What values do they share? The good news is that passions and core commitments to clinical excellence are remarkably similar among many nurses. In theory, these mutual loyalties can lead to a deeply motivating shared vision. But in real life, *the words people use* to describe their values *and the ways in which they use their words* can completely mask their core beliefs. While many nurses are dedicated to excellence in patient care, for example, they can have vastly different ways of expressing that dedication. It can be difficult for leaders to recognize, let alone embrace, distinctly different versions of nursing values they hold dear. If this is true for you, are there ways to move beyond your communication biases? How can you listen more openly to others' ways of expressing values and emotion?

FRESH PERSPECTIVE

If I am a stranger visiting your team, what would I notice about the group's interaction? In what ways is the team working optimally, and in what ways is it functioning less well? How would your team members answer these questions? What do your answers tell you about your quest to inspire a shared vision?

HOPES AND OTHER VARIABLES

Are there other factors that will promote or prevent the success of your initiative? Would you benefit from other assistance and support as you move ahead? When and how will you involve other organizational stakeholders in your efforts?

What professional dreams do your team members have? What motivates them? Can their hopes be included in your collective vision?

After you have considered these questions, it is time to act. Your specific steps will depend on your unique circumstances, so I invite you to add to, select from, or customize the following suggestions.

First, identify the areas of alignment and misalignment within your team. If there are multiple challenges, select the highest-priority issues to address. If you find it difficult to choose just a few, pick the problems that will yield the greatest leverage—the "biggest bang for the buck"—when they are solved.

Next, if there is disenchantment or resistance (or both) in your ranks, formulate your strategy for handling it. Although unpleasant, this emotional reality can literally poison your success. Its impact must be acknowledged and managed. Then build on your commonalities, address your concerns, and develop a concrete action plan. Communicate with other organizational colleagues and elicit their support.

Now, move ahead! With your team, dream your dreams and create your vision. Articulate your strategy, your goals, and your plans for implementing the vision so it is achievable and sustainable. Identify milestones and occasions when the team will review progress. Select times when the group will celebrate successes and evaluate and adjust strategy.

While obvious, this last point deserves emphasis. In my practice, I continually encounter nurse leaders who are so pressed for time that they sacrifice what's important in the long run for what's pressing in the short run. This is understandable, but this habit has seriously undesirable consequences over time. In this case, your team will miss fertile opportunities to review and adjust so that the new vision can take hold.

Making time to learn, reflect, and celebrate is well worth the effort. The return on your investment is both quantitative and qualitative. Your measurable results will be better, and your team will also feel better about their efforts. Let's make no mistake; feelings matter when it comes to creating a better future. Remember, the task is to inspire a shared vision! Your team will appreciate you and your recognition of their opinions, time, talent and commitment to creating—and living—into a vision of which you are all proud.

29

Shining Eyes

Your team needs to transform. The team members are in the "doldrums"; given the organization's recent challenges, their resistance and lack of energy are understandable. But you feel that enough is enough, and you want them to get back to performing and excelling, individually and collectively. As their leader, what is your role in helping them do this?

Just before we boarded the plane for our Midwest destination, my colleague and I received the news: the 3-day retreat we were about to convene might be cancelled. The chief nursing officer (CNO) who hired us had heard rumors that her team was not going to come despite her careful planning. We didn't take it personally; she hadn't given them any details about the offsite session. But she had indicated that it was an opportunity to deepen their leadership skills and their cohesion as a team.

The CNO (Rhoda) was newly promoted to her position in this health system that had changed ownership, replaced the entire management team, and implemented new organizational processes all in rapid order. Rhoda had planned this offsite to support and bolster her team of 25 nurses and their managers. She was acutely aware that the team had absorbed and endured the organization's many changes, most of which were beyond their control. Although Rhoda expressed compassion for that experience, she was also concerned about their lack of ownership of their actions, their behaviors on the job, and the potential consequences to patient well-being.

As we waited at the airport, my colleague and I listened to Rhoda's concerns on the phone and explored her options. After considerable thought, Rhoda decided she wanted to go ahead with the retreat.

Much to everyone's surprise, we started the program the next day with the full complement of 25 nurse leaders and managers. That was the good news. The bad news was that although the team members were in their seats and "nice" enough, their body language and their faces told a different story. They appeared to be distrustful of the CNO and wary of us. At best, they seemed guarded; at worst, they seemed cynical and disengaged.

In their book, *Art of Possibility*, Rosamund and Benjamin Zander talk about "shining eyes," which they use as a metaphor for the "spark of possibility" when a person is enrolled in a new vision that is of his or her own making.[a] Rhoda's team members' eyes were not shining—far from it. If ever there was a situation that called for transformation, this was it.

As the first day progressed, the group started talking about how they saw the organization and their roles in it. They had many complaints, and they railed against a system that required new processes even as the accompanying back-office procedures were still under development. The team saw themselves as victims and assigned blame to everyone around them.

Although they listened to the CNO, they regarded her with skepticism. The team spoke with a unified voice. It was clear that through all their trials, they had become a close-knit community with formal and informal leaders firmly in place. The CNO was new to her role but she was well known by this team, and she was not in either leadership camp.

This aggrieved group had many reasons, some justified, for their feelings of powerlessness and blame. The team, the CNO, and us, as conveners, had our work cut out for us. As facilitators, we knew our roles and we knew that the team's long-term success could be achieved and sustained only by the participants and Rhoda.

So what did Rhoda do in the face of this significant challenge?
- Over the course of 3 days, *she clearly laid out her expectations for attendance, participation, and outcomes.* She invited the team members to speak their truth and to listen to one another with respect and without judgment. She supported them in creating explicit behavioral guidelines for the retreat. She stated that there would be no repercussions for what they discussed.

---

[a]Rosamund and Ben Zander. *The Art of Possibility*. Boston, MA: Harvard Business School Press; 2000.

- *She explained that her commitment to this retreat represented an investment in each of them and in the team as a whole.* She told them that she had faith and confidence in them; she demonstrated empathy and support without dwelling on grievances for situations that were over, done, or beyond their control.
- *She stayed in the room, left her phone in her purse, and listened far more than she spoke.* She participated when her voice as leader was called for, but she did not dominate and capitulate when the group looked to her for "easy" answers that were the group's to create.
- *Although cordial and collegial, she was not overly friendly with us as facilitators.* She realized that the group could easily construe a cozy dynamic of aligned facilitators and the CNO as "them against us."

What did the team members do?

- *Despite rumors to the contrary, all of them showed up every day.* Many of them arrived 30 or more minutes early.
- *They listened more and more intently as the retreat unfolded.*
- *They were not afraid to speak up.* If they didn't agree with a facilitator or one of their team members, they said so.
- *They demonstrated a visible change between the end of the first day and the beginning of the second day.* The second morning provided a chance for them to voluntarily share their reactions to their work together so far. In response, one or two of the informal leaders offered surprisingly personal comments that demonstrated a sense of vulnerability and risk-taking. This created the space for others to do the same.
- *They replaced their sarcastic and edgy comments with more respectful ways of communicating.*

By the time the retreat was over, the team showed early signs of transformation. They realized that despite all the difficulties that were beyond their control, they still owned their roles and responsibilities. They considered what parts of their problems were of their own making. They shifted their focus from the finger-pointing of the past to the possibilities for the future. They developed action plans and accepted responsibility for implementing those plans in concert with the CNO and other appropriate team members.

Although the real test of the outcomes lies in their long-term success, this group is on its way to becoming a very different kind of a team. They were certainly bonded before the program, but their previously unchecked behavior brought out the worst in everyone and in the team as a whole. In contrast, their openness during the retreat allowed them to practice being a different kind of community, one that demonstrates respect even while disagreeing and one that is focused on ownership and positive change.

At the end of the third day, amid their touching appreciations for one another and the CNO for creating the conditions for their success, their eyes were truly shining. They reflected brighter images of one another and their hope and commitment to create a better future for their team, their organization, and their patients.

30

The Hidden Power of the Team Leader

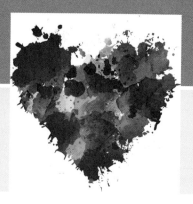

What is your effect on your team members? Do you know the impact of your actions, words, and beliefs on them? This is a story about an otherwise good leader's unintentionally limiting influence on her team. It is a tale about the consequences of this leader's restrictive language and beliefs, and how they kept her team from reimagining and embracing a compelling vision of what was possible.

Recently I coached a team of well-respected nurse leaders. We had embarked on a leadership development initiative to increase their effectiveness as individuals and as a group. We were well into a candid review of the team's concerns and opportunities when one of the prominent group leader said, "It would be nice if we could do that, but we can't. Remember, the box we are in is very small."

She was referring to the numerous systems and complexities in which they operate. She was talking about the stands taken by other senior leaders, their board of directors, their organizational policies and politics, and layers of regulations and accreditation criteria.

While some team members may have questioned her statement, most took it literally. This leader's belief that "the box is very small" created or solidified a reality for the rest of the team.

Without some type of intervention, from that moment forward this team might have acted on the belief that "this box is very small." That collective certainty would create a tight boundary around their possibilities and future achievements.

Here's the issue. Was this statement really true, either partially or completely? Either way, how much latitude did this team have to effect change, do things differently, and implement new and better systems and ideas? What responsibility did members of this team have to respectfully question this assertion?

Listen carefully to the words and their effect. "The box we are in is very small" sounds a lot like "We can't do that"

and "They won't let us." As professionals and nurse leaders, what obligation did the team have for speaking up for what they believed was right, even if it was outside the box? Was it their collective duty to take responsible risks and stand up for what they believed?

Under what circumstances do you find yourself saying the equivalent of "the box is very small"? Do you hear yourself saying, "We can't" and "They won't let us" more than you would like? If you answer "no" to these questions, congratulations! If you answer "yes," please keep reading.

What if the team operates in a bigger box than they think? What if the team can reshape the box? What was stopping them from seeing and seizing the opportunities they actually had? Here are some possibilities.

1. **We believe stories that are only partially true.** Stories are central to the perpetuation of our culture at all levels. But—and this is a truism—not all stories are of equal value or equally true. We all know this, but in some circumstances, we treat stories as if they are and will be completely true now and in the future. This occurs when such assertions resonate enough or when they are spoken by leaders we believe in.

2. **As leaders, we do not always examine the accuracy of our words.** This is important; the stories we tell about our organizations and ourselves are not always valid. Are we intentionally lying? No. Most of us are well-meaning, intelligent, fast-moving individuals, and we make assessments and draw conclusions because it is our responsibility to do so. We must make snap judgments on the basis of available information. We mix that information with our beliefs. Usually, our rapid response serves us and our organizations well—*except when the statements we make are partially false and inappropriately limiting.*

3. **We are not comfortable with taking risks.** Literature tells us that it is important for leaders to take risks. Nothing would change if we perpetually stayed with old ways. Every reader knows this. But when it comes to

actually taking risks, nurse leaders self-report that they often loathe taking risks. We are not comfortable challenging the size of the box.

4. **It can be easier to "play small."** Leaders can grow tired of leading with heart, that is, standing up for their beliefs, taking the high road, and working with others to implement new ways of doing and thinking. It is a tough task. It can be particularly draining if others create roadblocks, say "no," and are otherwise unsupportive. Leaders can lose their passion, energy, and enthusiasm for the good fight. The problem is that the good fight is the reason most of us signed up for this field and these roles. "They won't let us" becomes a very costly story. It robs us of our energy and robs others of their best contributions.

INCREASE VS. LIMIT THE POSSIBILITIES

So what do we do? How do we address self-limiting beliefs and statements that limit others too? How do we create stories that are "right-sized" rather than too small?

1. *Spend time with people who think differently.* They are all around you. They are in different disciplines, they are younger, they are older, and they are in fields other than health care. Those who are different are probably right there in your own team. Seek them out. Listen generously.

2. *Take risks that are worthwhile.* If you are not comfortable taking calculated risks, practice. Start small. Role-play. Think about the worst that can happen and plan accordingly. Remember and appreciate times when you have taken risks and succeeded.

3. *Challenge your own assumptions.* Think carefully about how accurate your beliefs are, especially if they limit you and others. If you doubt your ability to self-assess, talk with someone you trust. Review your ideas. Listen to yourself and ask yourself whether you really believe what you are saying. Reflect out loud with a friend, colleague, family member, or coach. Ask these other people to provide you feedback or to ask questions that will help clarify your thoughts, expand your views, and speak from a place of possibility.

4. *Challenge the assumptions of others.* In the story above, nobody challenged the statement offered by the leader because they respected and liked her. But we do a disservice to the team, the leader, and our organization when we do not question. There are ways to challenge assumptions with respect. For instance, one of them could have said, "Laura, I see exactly what you mean by that. Can we figure out a way to pursue this anyway?" What if we…"

5. *Ask questions.* Some effective risk takers begin by asking genuine questions. Their questions invite others to reexamine what they are saying. In the story above, for example, a team member might have asked, "Are there areas of opportunity for us despite this?" or "Maybe the box is bigger than we think. Remember when we took a risk and we succeeded, even though we were sure they would shoot us down?" These behaviors are worth trying. They can help all of us be more effective, and the reward is great. We can make more significant contributions, and we can act from a fuller version of our own power and strength.

31

The 70% Team

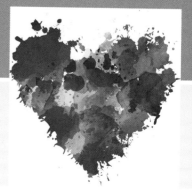

This team is functioning poorly. Its members have suffered multiple losses through reorganization and reassignments. As a result, they have lost trust in the organization and even in each other. They no longer can be counted on to follow through on their collective commitments, and they have a poor reputation with the rest of the organization. What can this team do to restore itself?

Recently, I was invited to work with a team of directors of clinical services in a successful, medium-sized health system. When I met with these nine leaders for the first time, I was impressed by each member's apparent competence and commitment. Despite their individual strengths, however, their results as a team were seriously lacking.

I was called in by the team leader to explore why the team was not performing well. Their individual assets suggested that they could be an excellent team, but by their own admission, they were not. Just one example was their ability to devise great team strategies when they were together but their failure to execute these strategies when they were apart. Once their meetings were over, each team member returned to her own department and ran her own show without regard for their collective decisions. The team members and others came to understand that their word—as a team—was not to be trusted in their own group or by others in the hospital.

In our first group meeting, it was clear that the team had a story to tell, and they were eager to share it. Like many nurse leaders, they had experienced a major reorganization. In that process, this team's previously private meetings were opened for others to attend, and the purpose of the meetings changed from information sharing and confidential conversation to tactical decision-making with others, often without advance notice and needed facts. Consequently, the team members found themselves reacting quickly and often negatively in these meetings. They felt like victims of the new organizational structure and

process. They said *no* to requests far more often than they said *yes*. They felt that their private time had been taken from them. Finally, they believed they had earned a bad reputation throughout the rest of the organization; others saw them as unhelpful and difficult.

As I reflected on our conversation, several themes emerged:

1. The team had a negative experience of itself. As a result, the team seemed to be unconsciously sabotaging its own power. For example, instead of asking for advance information to be better informed, the team continued to react, saying *no* because they were not prepared to make a different decision.

2. The team members did not hold each other accountable when they failed to honor team agreements or broke their commitments to one another. The team could describe this dysfunctional behavior very clearly to me, yet they could not recall any instance of discussing it at the time team agreements were violated.

3. The team members viewed themselves as victims; they had developed a strong belief that they were at the mercy of the decisions made by others and that they had no recourse to change those decisions or act on their own behalf.

4. The team experienced numerous losses during the reorganization. They lost team members, and as they perceived it, they lost the opportunity to make decisions that affected how they worked together. They also lost the chance to meet privately and to reflect together on organizational changes that affected their work, staff, and relationships. They also experienced the loss of the collegial regard and their due respect.

Whether your team displays any of these symptoms or has these particular concerns, there are points to learn from this particular situation. What can a team that is not functioning optimally do to turn itself around? How can such a team realize its full potential rather than just 70%?

In order for this team to move forward, they need to reimagine and let go of their experience of their recent past. As they eagerly described their history, they shared a story that had a flavor of "they did us wrong" and "they don't understand us." Although those feelings are understandable, holding onto them is not helping this team. It is highly unlikely that their colleagues will apologize for a clumsy reorganizational change strategy, and it is even less likely that anyone will say that the team was right. We all know that an approach that conveys a "woe is me" attitude is not attractive, compelling, or effective for us as individuals. It is even less effective when teams adopt this stance. When the team can process and let go of its past, it will be ready to move on.

In their stories, I could hear deep commitment and a wonderful set of values that could guide this team to greater accomplishment and service to their patients. I could see hints of the preferred future they imagined for themselves. As the team moves on, it can recognize and harness the strength of its passion and competence. The team members and their leader have the opportunity to create a truly compelling vision to pull them forward.

Once the team has a future vision that captures the best of their minds and hearts, they can create a strategy to execute that vision. The details of their strategy might include some or all of the following:

- *Mending relationships with individuals and groups that have been affected by the team's recent actions.*
- *Creating guidelines or rules of engagement so that the team has stated expectations for how it will operate going forward.* These could be as simple as showing up for meetings on time and listening to one another to understand rather than to agree. The rules of engagement could also include ways in which the team members want to hold one another accountable for following through on their commitments.
- *Assessing and addressing team learning needs such as conflict management or communication skills.*
- *Exploring the challenge of team collaboration.* The team needs to understand what is preventing its members from working together in a collaborative fashion after team decisions are made. Does the team know how to collaborate? What does effective collaboration look like for the leader and team members?
- *Candidly discussing the state of trust between and among team members.* If there are concerns about trust, it is likely that the team will continue to be dysfunctional to some degree. If trust has been violated, the team needs to understand what happened. The team can develop a set of guidelines that will allow its members to honestly dialogue and resolve past issues.
- *After the team has developed its vision and strategy, it will want to develop and implement an action plan.* They will want to keep track of their progress and evaluate and perhaps modify their actions as they go forward.

By taking these and similar steps, this team will restore its power and potency. Over time, others in the organization will recognize that the team is operating in a new and more effective way. Rather than operating at 70% of its ability, this team will be operating at full capacity. The team members will experience the significant benefits of working more closely, and patients and the health system will reap the rewards of a leadership team that excels.

Leading Change

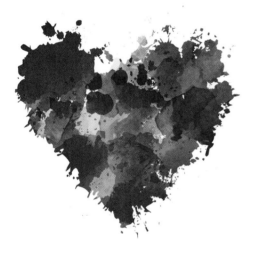

Thriving nurse leaders must be skilled at managing and implementing change. You know this, but are you as proficient with change management as you would like to be? How do you respond when rapidly shifting demands are placed on you, your coworkers, and your limited resources?

This section addresses how to manage change when it's happening quickly in your organization and all around you. It also focuses on how you can manage your coworkers when change is required and they are not ready. Finally, the section reviews how to approach change when it is you who is moving on.

32

Managing Too Much Change

Is there such a thing as too much change in an organization? Intuitively and experientially we know the answer is yes, but that doesn't stop change from occurring at a feverish pace. Here are strategies for what to do and what not to do when your organization is going through a large-scale change that significantly affects you and your staff.

Is there such a thing as too much change?

Most of us would say "yes." But, so what? Nurse leaders at all levels of any system must manage the amount of organizational change that is present, whether we think it is too much or not.

Recently, I was asked to work with a team of exceptional nurse leaders who were experiencing many significant changes in their organization. These changes included some that they could control and some that were uninvited and beyond their control, such as moving into a new facility, preparing for critical recertification visits, and implementing numerous staff changes and promotions.

To add to their already full plates, their chief nursing officer (CNO) recently resigned to pursue an outstanding opportunity. The remaining team members understood and supported that decision; most believed that they were well prepared to move ahead, even though the CNO had been a significant contributor to their organization's success. Still, they had a lot of feelings about the loss of their leader. They also felt anxious about who their new boss would be and what additional changes she or he would initiate.

To help endure these transitions, the organization's remaining senior leaders decided to elevate about half of the nursing leadership team to larger roles. Those individuals were given new titles, along with the label "interim"

(so the new CNO could decide whether to make the promotions permanent).

When I visited this facility, I encountered leaders who, to a person, were committed to patients and outstanding patient care. But when we drilled down just one level, I found other similarities that were disturbing:

- Most of these leaders looked defeated and reported feeling exhausted and overwhelmed.
- Their schedules were beyond full. Days were often 12 or more hours long. The leaders were meeting their usual commitments and also attending many other meetings required by the upcoming move.
- Most leaders had still more meetings to attend as a result of new responsibilities and positions. Finally, I discovered that information about the departure of the CNO and the temporary promotions had been promptly shared with some team members but not others. They were also concerned that the senior leaders were playing favorites with the team members. Consequently, the whole team was starting to distrust the organization's senior leaders. On the whole, the team's behaviors, feelings, and attitudes belied their historical power. I had worked with them before, and I knew that they could operate at full-throttle energy and efficacy. This time, however, they were disheartened and overwhelmed. The way in which they "showed up" as individuals and as a group suggested a story of deep fatigue, defeat, and too little time to absorb the following:
- New learning and the responsibilities of their new jobs and reporting relationships.
- The uncertainty of how long their jobs and reporting relationships would last.

- Unclear expectations about what to accomplish and how far to go with their own ideas with their interim roles and interim bosses.
- The challenges of leading a significant organizational initiative (the move).
- The need to think and act strategically in the face of so many operational demands.
- Uncertainty about a new and unknown CNO.

WHEN SUSTAINED BEST EFFORTS ARE REQUIRED

If you similarly find yourself in the midst of orchestrating major organizational change and requiring the extraordinary efforts of your leaders, what best practices can you use?

- *Encourage self-care.* If your team members can't identify their true priorities amidst a long list of "musts," help and encourage them to sort them out. Give them parameters and offer them feedback so that they can reduce their list of must-do activities.
- *Understand that human beings can become unhappy when major change occurs* and they don't understand or feel that they have complete information and a say in their future.
- *Realize that senior leaders are more efficient at leading change when they communicate those changes,* including what is known and not known, over and over again. Even if leaders think they have already said what is happening, they need to communicate their knowledge again and again. Successful change leaders share their news in multiple venues: one-on-one sessions and staff meetings, town halls, newsletters, e-mails, etc.
- *Include opportunities for two-way dialogue* to signal your openness and respect and to promote understanding and trust.
- *Do not ask selected others to keep secrets*, because it can erode trust and breed rumors. Leaders and staff who are not in the know are often aware that there are secrets, even if they don't know the specifics. When people know something is happening and suspect that it will impact them, they become fearful and open to unfounded rumors. Some will even make up stories to explain what they don't know or understand. In

the absence of authoritative information, those on the receiving end of rumors have no way of knowing what's true and what isn't. The bottom line: too many secrets destroy trust between leaders and the people who look up to them.

- *Be visible and demonstrate courage when there is news to share.* Be honest and straightforward about it, even if it's bad news. People hearing garbled or incomplete truths can become angry and confused. They can slide into inaction, depression, disempowerment, and fatigue.
- *Be thoughtful about temporary titles and reporting relationships.* If you do establish them, set parameters and be available to address questions and concerns for the duration of these assignments. At the beginning, specify whether you want them to assume caretaker roles or act in more substantial ways. Clarify what you mean by either or a mix of the two approaches.
- *Create big spaces for your leaders to fill even if their roles may not be long term.* Don't inadvertently let your leaders fall into a minimally productive, "let's wait and see" mode, even if their future bosses are unknown. Give them stretch goals for the near term. Allow them to focus on what the organization needs. Let them continue to realize their potential and be successful.

If you are a leader who is on the receiving end of a great deal of change and transition, remember to focus on your own well-being, as well as your effectiveness as a leader. Review the list above; if you need more information or feedback in any of the listed areas, ask for it even if your manager doesn't initiate the conversation.

Remember who you are as a leader with mastery and heart. Even if the circumstances create huge unknowns for your future, remember yourself at your best. Think about what you do when you are at your best and identify what you can do in your current situation to bring out your best again.

Ask yourself what opportunities the uncertainty offers you. If you can't think of any, ask yourself again. Keep asking until you start to see some benefits in your less-than-ideal situation. Remember that, even if your circumstances are not what you want, *you* are in control of how you think about and manage yourself and others.

33

Readiness and Reinforcement Matter

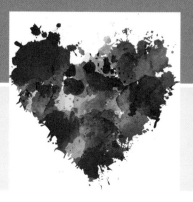

Change is afoot, and readiness and long-term support are necessary for it to take hold. What are the consequences when leaders don't reinforce the behaviors, attitudes, and practices that are essential for sustaining change? Are you ready to back your coworkers as they adjust to new circumstances? Here are some factors to consider.

Let's consider two scenarios. In the first, Karen is a nurse with 25 years of management and leadership experience. She wants a new job so that she can use her full complement of leadership skills. She has all the right credentials, yet after 2 years of looking she has been unable to secure a new position.

In the second scenario, Ramona is a vice president in a large health care system. She has eight nurse manager direct reports, and she recently terminated one of them, Cindy, because of Cindy's lack of follow-through and her unwillingness to be accountable. Cindy's poor performance affected patients, staff nurses, and Ramona's other direct reports.

Once Cindy was gone, Ramona decided to devote scarce financial resources to a team retreat. Her planning was meticulous, and her goals were clear: acknowledge the hard work and success of the remaining managers, rebuild morale, and instill greater accountability into the team. The retreat was more successful than Ramona expected, yet several weeks later, Ramona's direct reports had even lower morale than before, and accountability had not improved.

What do these two nurse leaders have in common? Karen and Ramona are not taking the "readiness factor" into account.

What is the readiness factor? Readiness refers to our *intrapersonal* self-awareness and management, and our *interpersonal* ways of relating to others. Intrapersonal readiness means that we consciously acknowledge and manage our own emotional state. Interpersonal readiness means we are aware of how we are relating to others and what our impact is.

How does readiness apply to Karen, the nurse leader with the experience and credentials for a new leadership role? People who interact with Karen describe her as bitter and whiny; they feel uncomfortable in her presence. They say that she has an attitude of entitlement when she talks about her current employer. Karen thinks she is prepared for another role that is more challenging, and on paper she is. But discerning hiring managers are not selecting her because she speaks so negatively about her current job. They can see that Karen has not done the personal work that is required to successfully move on.

What about Ramona? The retreat went beautifully and the immediate results far surpassed anything she and the team could have imagined. However, Ramona was not ready to reinforce those results in ways that mattered to her team. The team had experienced what they described as a trauma with Cindy, the former team member. Although they discussed these difficult events during the retreat, the team needed Ramona's attention and support *after the retreat* to heal the past and to sustain their fragile new direction.

Ramona had not equipped herself to do what was required when the retreat was over. She had not considered that a successful retreat would mean a shift in her focus too. She intended for the retreat to change the team's morale and behavior, but she did not consider her impact and role in supporting the change she wanted to see.

Ramona was not ready to do anything different after the retreat. In fact, she took a 2-week vacation right after the gathering. When she returned, the post-retreat glow had passed, and the team's low morale had returned in a more virulent form. Why? The team believed that they had tried and failed to fix their problems. As a result, they were even more demoralized.

These two examples show us that our lack of attention to readiness and reinforcement can be quite costly. Karen is meeting potential employers who are turned off by her negativity, and she is losing her professional standing in her community. Health care teams that could use Karen's expertise are not benefiting from it. Ramona spent scarce dollars and time on a retreat, yet the process actually harmed the team because they could not sustain their fragile new beginning without the post-retreat presence and support of their leader. Consequently, the team members felt defeated and unsuccessful.

What went wrong? Neither Ramona nor Karen reflected on these critical questions: Am I (or are we) ready to be successful? *What it will take to get ready? What is my (our) emotional condition, and how am I coming across right now? What is my impact on others? Am I prepared to take care of myself and/or support others so I and we can move on and sustain success?*

Most of us do ask ourselves reflective questions when we contemplate needs or opportunities, but we concentrate on the required skill-based competencies and front-end resources. We are not as diligent when contemplating whether we and others are emotionally prepared to move ahead, and we do not always attend to what is needed *after* a change, a promotion, or an initiative has taken place.

RECOGNIZING READINESS

A lack of readiness may look like resistance, confusion, anger toward others, or passive/aggressive behavior. For example, Karen exhibits whininess and an inability to let go of the negative emotions about her current situation. That's her story and she's sticking to it.

When individual contributors and teams are not ready, they may agree to proceed with a new plan or idea, but they are not fully committed. They may subtly, and unconsciously, sabotage the project. They may have questions, but they may not ask them. They may withdraw but still show up in body, but not in spirit. They may do what is required, but they will not extend discretionary effort.

By contrast, when we and others are ready for new challenges, we display some or many of these qualities:
- We are curious and energized by what is new.
- We are motivated to achieve fresh goals and greater success.
- We are open to feedback and we are not defensive when we receive it.
- We anticipate, provide, ask for, or receive support when we and others need it.

- We are open and truthful with ourselves and others.
- We are ready to be challenged with new material, new people, and new opportunities.
- We take risks when they are appropriate.

THE LEADER'S ROLE

A leader has three key responsibilities when it comes to readiness for and reinforcement of change:
1. *Assess the readiness of direct reports. In addition to monitoring the aforementioned qualities, leaders will also consider:*
   - Clinical, administrative, or other technical training required to take on the new assignment
   - Interest in moving ahead in the direction the assignment suggests
   - Ability or inability to let go (e.g., displaying an excessive attachment to a peer group or "the way things were")
   - Being clear or stuck in a victim mentality (e.g., demonstrating a strong emotional connection to perceived wrongs done to themselves or others)
   - Commitment to professional growth and advancement, personally and organizationally
   - Values alignment with other organizational leaders
   - Sufficient self-awareness to reflect on and manage one's own problems and limitations
2. *Provide appropriate resources to prepare others for new challenges and responsibilities. These include:*
   - Vehicles and time for training
   - Support through coaching, mentoring, peer groups, or similar means
   - Sufficient lead time for the preparation to take hold
   - Recognition of small wins and big successes
3. *Offer support before, during, and after the initiative so progress can be sustained.*

Although all nurses are not candidates for better jobs, more responsibility, and greater team effectiveness, many are. Once equipped with greater awareness of the readiness factor, nurse leaders can provide support, training, coaching, or other forms of preparation for their managers, staff, and themselves. The readiness factor operates under the radar in many situations. When we actively address it, all of us gain.

34

Understanding Resistance

Managing change requires that leaders understand resistance and the many forms it takes. You can be more skilled at working with resistance when you know why people resist. Often, it is because they believe they are losing something and they are grieving or angry about it. At times, people resist because they are deeply committed to a value that they perceive is threatened. How can you address loss, grief, and fear so that you and your colleagues can all move forward?

One reader is a manager who wants to change her unit's culture, but she is encountering stubborn resistance. Another has a vocal employee who is negatively influencing others. The third reader wants to inspire nurses to help them reengage.

What do these nurse leaders have in common? Each has the chance to develop rapport and renewed commitment with those who are resisting.

Is this a desirable outcome every time? No. Sometimes it is appropriate for the manager to get tough and/or for the employees to move on. But in these instances, let's assume that each of these leaders can create a positive outcome that engages nearly everyone. Let's say the unit culture *is* in need of change and that most staff members perceive this need. Let's say that the disaffected employee was once a star performer. Let's say that until recently, the nurses were satisfied with their positions.

How do we approach others when they resist our direction? One common leadership strategy is to become more determined. We hold meetings and retreats in which we provide more data and tell compelling stories. We offer supporting evidence, and we invoke the organizational mandate. No matter what the particulars are, our strategy is to provide more information so others will better understand our position. *We believe that more data will persuade people.*

A second approach is to dig in and insist. Rather than the more subtle educational campaign described above, we move forward with a heavier hand. This is also known as the "this is the way we are going to do it" approach. We know this is not the best leadership choice, but we may opt for it anyway. We might be frustrated. We might be out of time. We might simply need to shut down disagreement and move ahead.

Any of these approaches can be successful. Yet, choosing these paths too frequently can limit our learning and may stem from an *emotional* truth about us—*we are resisting the resistance.* We simply don't want to hear the complaining or experience the difficulty of talking with people who are not signing up for our point of view. The good news is that this reaction is entirely human!

So, is it possible to be human and to experience our own reluctance to engage with negativity but still move beyond these instincts? Can we explore the wisdom, if any, that resistance offers us?

I had a wise mentor who once divided "resisting complainers" into two camps. Both types, she said, are truly committed people. The first are those who are committed to complaining! Regrettably for them and for others, these people are perpetually unhappy and continually vocal. It's the second category that holds lessons for us. These are the people who are committed to something they fear losing. In nursing, it may be a professional value they hold dear. It may be a nursing practice they feel is threatened or compromised.

Let's reconsider our leaders' challenges. The first is facing stubborn opposition from those on the unit who do not want change. What if this manager were to momentarily set aside her own negative emotional response to what they are saying and how they are saying it? What if she were to create a safe environment in which they could honestly explore their concerns? What if she approached them with an open mind and genuine willingness to listen?

If she were to do this, she could learn a lot. It is possible she will hear that they are afraid of losing something. Perhaps it is their autonomy. Perhaps they are concerned about giving up habits the organization once tolerated but can no longer afford.

If she is able to listen openly, she may hear valuable kernels of truth. This does not mean she will agree with *all* their points. But she may agree with and *focus on* some of them. She may hear concerns she too would have if she were in their position. She may hear ways in which the organization has, perhaps inadvertently, enabled them to develop these views.

Listening differently may help her realize that the organization is partially responsible for their concerns. She may even decide to publicly state the organization's share of accountability for the past while maintaining the need to move forward.

As they discuss their concerns, she may hear values she and they *mutually* share. She could build on these mutual values and skillfully shift the conversation from what they don't want to what they *do* want. Together, they can craft a solution that will build on what is important to *all* of them. Together, they can move ahead.

What if the other two leaders were to have similar conversations? There is no question that this is courageous work, but it is immensely worthwhile and can begin with several simple steps. First, these leaders would honor but not succumb to their own unpleasant experience of resistance. They would momentarily set aside their feelings of "being right." They would assess these individuals. What types of resisters are they? Are they committed to complaining, or are they committed to values they feel are compromised or threatened? Are they fearful of change? What is behind their fear? Has the organization in some way contributed to their past experience and current beliefs?

A leader's private assessment cannot reveal the answers to all these questions, but it can steer her in the right direction. A courageous leader can explore such concerns with curiosity, an open mind, and an open heart. If our leader is able to listen with genuine interest, she may be able to identify values they *all* hold closely. New solutions can surface. At the very least, new understanding and greater trust will emerge.

35

What Does "No" Really Mean?

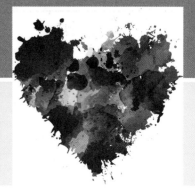

You find yourself with a staff full of resisters. What should you do? There are three types of resistance, according to Rick Maurer in his book, Beyond the Wall of Resistance.[a] Read on to discern what types of resisters are in your audience and what strategies will be successful with them.

Not long ago, my colleague Jennifer visited a hospital that had engaged our team to work with their nursing leaders. Jennifer was convening a voluntary "brown bag" luncheon to check in with the program participants. She also promised to review a key program activity as the meeting ended.

Jennifer enjoyed good relationships with these leaders, and this meeting was no exception. They began with a lively discussion of their most recent challenges. The economy was playing havoc with hospital finances and their individual budgets. This forum gave the leaders the chance to speak their minds candidly and in heartfelt ways. They faced significant leadership trials, and over the coming months they wanted help to keep their staff members engaged, even as they themselves were anxious about economic uncertainties.

A few minutes before the meeting ended, Jennifer shifted the dialogue to a key program activity that was planned for the next several months. She spoke with the same easy, honest tone that had prevailed previously. No sooner had she started speaking than she noticed a decided shift in the room. The participants, who had been completely engaged just minutes before, fell silent. Despite Jennifer's attempts to make a smooth transition, she could not reignite a compelling conversation. Instead, she faced people who appeared bored, complacent, and unavailable. They all seemed to be saying, "I am not interested in what you are saying, and I am resisting it completely."

There are many leaders who experience circumstances like Jennifer's. What do we do when we find ourselves before an audience of "resisters"? Many leaders say that their emotions kick in right away, and visibly or invisibly,

they react as if their good ideas have been summarily rebuked. They may feel that they have been rejected personally. Egos become ensnared, and stated or unstated conflict blossoms. Emotions are stirred, and the leader's effectiveness is compromised.

RECOGNIZE THE THREE TYPES OF RESISTANCE

So what should we do when we encounter resistance? One good option is to mentally review a model that Rick Maurer describes on his website[b] and in his book, *Beyond the Wall of Resistance*. Maurer talks about three levels of resistance:

- *"I don't get it."* When people don't understand something, they can demonstrate resistance in various ways. They may hide their lack of comprehension or appear confused, angry, stubborn, or uninterested.
- *"I don't like it."* People may understand a proposal quite well, but they don't like it. As leaders, it is important to remember that when people don't like what we want to do, perhaps it is because our new way forward represents a threat or loss to them.
- *"I don't like you."* In this case, for whatever reason, the personal relationship between the leader and those resisting is damaged. There are many possible causes. Two options are that the leader has not listened or the other individuals think that the leader does not care about their viewpoints.

How can Jennifer use this information to move through the resistance she experienced?

- Based on the evidence before and after the meeting, Jennifer determined that her personal relationship with the other leaders was intact.
- Jennifer concluded that these leaders exhibited a combination of two forms of resistance: "I don't get it"

---

[a]Maurer R. *Beyond the Wall of Resistance: Unconventional Strategies That Build Support for Change.* Austin, TX: Bard Press; 1996.

[b]The resources you need to lead change ... without resistance. Maurer and Associates website. http://www.beyondresistance.com. Accessed December 26, 2009.

and "I don't like it." Some participants may not have seen the relevance between the project she was talking about and the serious leadership challenges they were facing. Therefore, it was up to Jennifer to ensure that the assigned task could encompass their concerns and to communicate how that could happen.

- Still others may have been clear on what Jennifer proposed and wanted no more information. They had already decided that Jennifer's task was off-target and irrelevant. Again, it was up to Jennifer to ensure that she was successful in engaging them and hearing their concerns. She also needed to work together with the leaders to ensure that the task was accomplished while simultaneously meeting their own legitimate needs.

What can we learn from Jennifer's circumstances?

1. *Ignoring the urge to respond instantly is smart.* When we are in the action of leadership and experience resistance, it is tempting to decide quickly what the resistance means and implement a solution immediately. But, if we can slow our responses down even for a moment, we can consider what that "no" really means. Taking a moment to reflect gives us more options than going forward with a knee-jerk response that is off-target.

2. *Resistance provides us with important feedback.* We are wise to pay attention to resistance and the message it contains. We may not agree with any part of the message or choose to validate it in any way, but it is still important to consider its meaning.

3. *Resistance has many faces.* Confusion, denial, sabotage, soliciting the support of others who sympathize, engaging in passive-aggressive behavior, and needing more and more information—all these are potential symptoms of resistance.

4. *We can correctly diagnose the type of resistance we are experiencing.* Do people really need more information? What if they have enough information to know that they don't like our "solution" because they don't perceive its value or relevance?

5. *There are nearly always (at least) two sets of needs operating–theirs and ours.* In this instance, Jennifer realized that the participants needed to be heard: how were they going to be good leaders in such a tough climate? Her own needs called for crafting a successful leadership development activity. She could be successful easily by accommodating both sets of needs.

Jennifer reexamined the project with the team at their next meeting. What could have become immovable group resistance eventually transformed into a palpable commitment to an engaging peer-learning activity. The group went on to truly embrace Jennifer's "project," especially when they personally experienced the spot-on leadership support it generated.

Their initial resistance relaxed into acceptance, generosity, and mutual support because the group was willing to reconsider their initial reactions, and because their leader Jennifer recrafted her approach to directly and honestly address the group's needs and concerns.

36

Managing by Accident

Nurse managers and leaders are not always in their roles because they chose them. At times, organizational change thrusts nurses who have been happy at the bedside into leadership roles, supposedly "temporarily." Yet, what's temporary often becomes permanent, even when these leaders resist because they don't want these positions. What is the best way to work with managers who have been "drafted" into their roles?

Consider your team for a moment. Whether you are the nurse leader, team supervisor, or team member, think about how the nurse manager (you?) became the nurse manager. Did you or she have a plan to move into that role? Or did you arrive in the job by accident?

Now, consider other nurse managers you know. How did they arrive in those positions? Did they carefully guide their careers to this destination?

If we could take a real-time poll of readers, we would probably learn that many nurse managers take on the role without a plan to become a manager. In fact, many managers might have had absolutely no interest. They might say something like this direct quote from an accidental manager, "One day I was asked if I would take this job temporarily. That was 2 ½ years ago!"

I feel confident about my prediction because I have heard this and similar stories many times from nurse leaders and managers. It is particularly compelling to hear these tales when they are revealed publicly, with other nurse managers close by. Clearly, these inadvertent managers resonate with one another as they share their respective accounts of their "recruitment." Lots of spontaneous laughter fills the room as they describe the many ways their hiring supervisors asked them to fill these roles.

As bonding among the members of a group of accidental managers occurs, the stories grow richer and deeper. Themes like these emerge:
- I love being a bedside nurse, and I miss my old life.
- I never wanted to be a manager. My boss and the chief nursing officer (CNO) have lifestyles that I don't want.

- This is a difficult job. I often agree with my old friends on the unit, but I have to act like I believe something else.
- I don't know how to do this job. I was put in the position many months ago, and I have still not had any training.
- This job is very stressful.

As leaders, it is important for us to realize that we may have a managerial team that includes a number of inadvertent "draftees" who feel this way. It is in our best interest to treat these individuals with the respect they deserve as they temporarily or permanently do the heavy lifting that management requires.

SUPPORTING MANAGEMENT "DRAFTEES"

What can we do to demonstrate our respect, support, and interest in their welfare?
- *We need to listen carefully.*
- *We need to offer them education and training.*
- *We need to ask open-ended, curious questions to find out how they are doing.*
- *We need to clearly understand, in their terms, what they believe they need to succeed.*
- *We must be available to them.*
- *We must create a safe relationship so that they are free to talk with us,* take reasonable risks, and feel comfortable as they grow into positions that they did not seek.
- *We need to earn their trust.*
- *We may need to offer them coaching or personal mentoring.*
- *We need to graciously allow these nurses to go back to bedside nursing if that is their preference* after we have taken these steps.

A recent example shows how pivotal these strategies can be. For about a year, Violet was a nurse manager "draftee" for a key service line at a large university medical center. She was asked to take on the role temporarily while the organization decided whether and how to fill the position permanently.

In a training program a couple of months ago, she came forward in a room full of nurse managers. She wanted to talk about her concern as a new, accidental manager. As Violet told her story, it was clear that her problem was so upsetting that she was ready to leave her job.

Violet said that her staff did not have the resources they needed to do their work. She felt strongly that they didn't have what was required to produce quality outcomes and satisfactory patient experiences. She had asked her boss for these resources on several occasions, but her boss never said yes. She summed up her current situation as following:
- She didn't believe she was making a clear "business" case for her manager.
- She didn't believe her manager was really listening to her.
- She didn't believe her manager was concerned about or understood what it takes for bedside nurses to create top-quality patient outcomes and satisfaction.

Our group of classroom listeners could not have been more empathetic. They leaned in to hear Violet, and as they did, she received palpable support and many suggestions. The faculty member guiding the session invited Violet to consider what her next step would be if she were to stay on the job a little longer. She said she would go back to her manager one more time.

At the invitation of the faculty member, Violet rehearsed that next conversation with her manager. After a few rounds of practice, she said that she was prepared and ready to meet her manager "one last time."

As she reflected on her experience when the session ended, Violet described what had just happened in the room:
- She had the experience of being listened to and supported.
- She learned that she was still committed to the organization and wanted to try once more to ask for what she needed.

- She found that being honest and practicing with someone who will listen and give good feedback was very helpful.
- She learned to hear herself and to restate things that don't come out right the first time.
- She learned that her approach doesn't have to be perfect right away and that, with practice and attention, it gets better.
- She learned that she doesn't have to take everyone's suggestions for how to handle her challenges. She learned to listen with discernment.

The next week, Violet returned to her institution and implemented her plan. Later, she told the program faculty what happened. In her own words, she was "truly shocked" by the outcome. Her manager not only gave Violet an immediate increase in resources but also offered to accompany her to a meeting with their mutual boss, the CNO. In the meeting, they would both make the case for even more resources for Violet's areas.

Violet was thrilled. Her victory is a success that many accidental managers can enjoy. The first step in Violet's newfound triumph involved the uncomplicated act of being heard. Simple as it is, it can be so difficult for time-starved leaders to find the time to listen, but it is so worth it. Giving these managers and potential future leaders our full attention and support is a win for all—the nurse manager, the patients, the organization, and all of us. Indeed, Violet's experience with this approach confirms that it is an important strategy for developing and retaining our best talent.

37

A Mentee's Lament

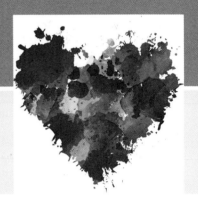

If you are lucky, you have had at least one wise mentor who has greatly influenced your growth as a leader. Invaluable as these individuals are, can you outgrow them? Yes, and if you do outgrow them, do you know how to respectfully manage this important relationship as it changes? As the mentee, are you ready to appreciate your mentor and then move on? As the mentor, can you support your mentee while s/he does this?

During our first meeting, Suze, a young nurse leader, appeared grounded, eager, filled with ambition, and clear about her goals. "I want to change the world," she announced. Her words and demeanor suggested that she is capable of doing just that, but she feels stalled in her current position. She described some of its limitations, and she also lamented the fact that she has no mentors.

Suze holds a regional-level service line post in a large health care entity. She enjoys considerable support among her contemporaries, and her written evaluations are outstanding. All the data indicate that Suze is a star. Many of her colleagues believe that she is capable of advancing to her organization's highest levels.

Although Suze holds an executive position in a critical functional area, she does not have organizational experience outside the regional office. Her immediate superior, Norma, brought Suze into the organization 5 years ago, and she has guided Suze's steady rise to prominence. Norma is a brilliant strategist and communicator, according to Suze, but she is also abrasive, difficult, impatient, and not well liked. People are afraid of her. Suze portrays their relationship as "Suze, good cop" and "Norma, bad cop."

Although Suze admires Norma and is grateful to her, it is clear that she is also ready to move. Even though Norma has served as a functional mentor to Suze, like many mentees, Suze does not and has not ever seen Norma in this light.

Suze has many job options in her organization. When she discusses these with Norma, Norma informs her of the negative consequences of each choice. In every opportunity, Norma finds a significant problem. As we talk further, a pattern emerges: Norma doesn't like any prospect that is beyond her own span of control and influence. Suze is aware that "leaving" Norma will be difficult. She realizes that Norma may experience her wish to move on as disloyal and "punish" her in some way.

Stepping back from the details, we see Suze as an outstanding young leader who has reached a turning point in her career and in her relationship with her supervisor. This part of Suze's journey is one that many of us experience—where once we were indebted to and enthralled with our supervisor or informal "mentor's" ways, those same qualities begin to chafe, even if just a bit. It's not that what we have learned is not useful, but it's that we are ready to go beyond it.

Suze's dilemma reveals insights into both mentor and mentee challenges when their most significant learning is behind them rather than before them. In this case, Norma's actions may be motivated by fear, whether conscious or unconscious. Perhaps Norma believes that Suze's departure will render her less effective. Perhaps she is concerned about what it will look like if a star "leaves her." Perhaps Norma is aware that if her poor behavior is exposed, her own career could stall.

At the same time, Suze is experiencing new facets of herself as a leader. She feels she has reached the limits of her ability to grow and learn from her mentor, yet she still values her mentor's brilliance and contribution. Suze may be afraid that she too will be less effective; what if she is not as successful without the guidance and protection of her boss? What does Suze do now?

- *First, she must realize that the responsibility for her growth as a leader ultimately rests with her, not her mentor.*
- *She can recognize that the relationship with her supervisor must change if she is to continue to develop and learn.*
- *She can acknowledge that implementing this change will require considerable personal courage.*
- *She can show compassion for herself.* Leaving the familiarity of a relationship with a significant mentor and entering into the unknown is challenging for anyone, especially a young leader who is venturing beyond a powerful force like Norma.
- *She can accept that making this change will alter the form and depth of the relationship with Norma, but it need not signal its end.*

Wise mentees consciously consider what they have learned from their mentors and whether and how they want to continue to relate to them. Even if a continuing relationship is not possible or desirable, the mentee can still let her mentor know the ways in which their relationship has been especially valuable.

If you relate more to the mentor's side of this story, here are some questions you can consider:

When a mentee or a favorite direct report is ready for challenges that are beyond what you can offer, how do you react?

1. *Do a strict and scrupulously honest personal accounting of how you relate to your mentee now.* If he or she has excelled within your area but would benefit from moving outside it, are you doing all you can to help and support the mentee so they can do that?

2. *If you feel a sense of vulnerability when a trusted lieutenant is about to leave, what steps can you take to address your personal needs?* How can you increase your safety while lessening your unintended dependence on your mentee?

3. *If you find yourself actively or passively deflecting a star's efforts to grow in new directions, what will it take for you to move past your resistance so you can offer your blessing and help?*

4. *If you believe he or she is about to make a mistake, can you give your mentee the benefit of your viewpoint while also letting her know that you still support her?*

Suze took her many options and the lessons of her mentor/mentee relationship to heart. She created criteria and ultimately selected a job that will give her needed experience in leading a key process redesign effort in a local acute care facility for 6 months. She can then return to her regional position if she wishes. Initially, Norma did not approve of this move, but Suze stood her ground. When Norma saw that Suze was proceeding anyway, she reframed Suze's decision and declared that she would "detail" Suze to do this same work in all of her facilities when Suze returns. Suze does not want to do this, and she is prepared to say no to Norma when that time comes.

As Suze prepares for her new role, she goes with Norma's blessing. Suze is leaving to deepen her experience and pursue her dream of changing the world. By moving courageously toward this new choice, Suze added a critical dimension to her personal power. Despite her supervisor's resistance, she devised a careful process for reviewing her options, deciding what to do and where to do it. She also decided what guidance to take with her and what guidance to leave behind.

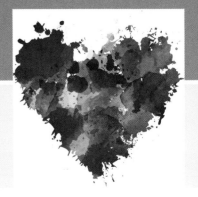

38

Meet the New Boss

You have a new boss. What will this mean for you? Sweeping organizational change happens a lot, and sometimes it includes leadership changes that affect you. Do you know how to support yourself during periods of uncertainty? As a masterful leader, you can take the reins rather than wait for events to be "done to you." You can be prepared to craft a strong relationship with your new boss, and you can also be ready to move on if your position is eliminated or it becomes untenable.

Long ago, the rock group "The Who" immortalized the line "Meet the new boss, same as the old boss."[a] Originally, these words symbolized the disappointment of a generation seeking, but not finding, large-scale change. Now, however, the prospect of no change is comforting to LuAnn, a seasoned vice president in a large health system on the West Coast.

Like many health care leaders, LuAnn is facing undefined, but certain, future budget constraints. She also has another challenge; her chief executive officer (CEO) is leaving. The current CEO brought her aboard, and he has championed her many successes during her 15-year tenure.

LuAnn is a nurse in her mid-50s. She anticipates working at least another decade; she loves her work, and she had planned to retire from her current position. Those around her would agree that she has thrived as steward of an organizational function that has enjoyed enthusiastic support from the CEO but tepid interest from other senior leaders.

LuAnn's nursing background infuses her with a genuine passion for her work, and she relishes her team's contribution to the well-being of patients and their families. Through both qualitative data and anecdotal experiences, LuAnn knows that her department makes a significant difference in the community.

Like many of us, LuAnn has her share of personal concerns, particularly as she and her family recover from some economic hardship. Still, she maintains a good deal of tangible success and is clear about how she does it—through hard work, a strong belief in her own values and those of the organization, her unwavering attention to the priorities of senior leadership, and her commitment to creating outstanding results that can be measured through both numbers and stories.

Now, LuAnn's organization is grappling with challenges that she believes will directly affect her position. In addition to having a potentially smaller or nonexistent budget and a new, unknown CEO, the organization recently shifted LuAnn's reporting relationship away from the retiring CEO. She now reports to an individual who does not share her passion for the work. In fact, her new boss may want to eliminate LuAnn's entire function, thereby achieving considerable cost savings for the organization.

Understandably, LuAnn is concerned that she might soon be out of a job. Actually, she is more than concerned; she is afraid. She admits that she has had many sleepless nights since she learned that the CEO was going to depart.

If you were LuAnn, how would you cope with your fear and uncertainty? How would you handle your concerns while still providing strong leadership for your department?

Let's look at what LuAnn actually did in these circumstances. To manage her anxiety and maintain her effectiveness, she employed five distinct strategies. She became conscious and intentional about selecting the strategy or strategies that would best serve her in specific situations.

1. ***She engaged a trusted advisor and discussed her feelings about all the changes that were occurring on her job.*** She also talked with friends, family, and some colleagues. She did not isolate herself, nor did she overexpose her feelings with inappropriate audiences. Her circle of trusted individuals helped her determine whether her fears were real and whether her predictions were likely to happen. Her openness and their input helped LuAnn focus on likely scenarios rather than potential but far-fetched possibilities.

[a]Townsend P. Won't get fooled again. On: Who's Next. Decca Records. 1971.

2. *She also reflected on the worst—the loss of her job.* She considered the impact upon herself and her family. She developed an interim plan that not only addressed their short-term needs but also created a viable bridge to long-term financial survival.

3. *She thought about what she would really like to do if the unthinkable occurred.* The first time she pondered this bleak prospect, she couldn't think of anything else she wanted to do. As time passed, however, her spirits lifted as she realized that even if the work were organized differently, she could still do what she most loves to do, perhaps even in her current organization. She also began to appreciate that other organizations would value her skills and experience too. She made a list of those places and prepared to research them if needed. The essence of this strategy is significant: *LuAnn decoupled herself from the form and structure of her current work and instead focused on her passions, the content, the impact, and importance of the work itself (versus its departmental home or her title).*

4. *With her trusted advisors, LuAnn discussed upcoming meetings in which the future of "her" services would be considered.* She worked on being clear about her role, her voice, and the position she would take in each of these meetings. At times, she concentrated on a particular high-stakes meeting's agenda and its attendees. She developed a meeting-specific approach to deploying her knowledge of her function, its benefits, and/or her point of view about her department's reason for being. In other words, she clarified whether she wanted to speak as an educator about the department or an advocate for its services or both. She sought feedback on her communication approach and style and the likely impact she would have. She was mindful of her role as a champion for the health system as a whole, not just her individual function. In every case, she made choices about how she wanted to present herself. She reminded herself to deal with her fear of losing her job *outside* the meetings so that she would not be overcome with emotions *during* them.

5. *In some cases, she literally practiced what she would say in stressful conversations in the larger management circle.* Sometimes she asked others to role-play so that she could run through her comments. Rehearsing allowed LuAnn to anticipate actual discussions, hear her own voice, and become more comfortable with potential conflict and challenges to her work or livelihood.

LuAnn's story illustrates that even without her champion CEO, she could sustain herself during seriously challenging times. She worked hard to manage her fear and the uncomfortable ambiguity in her life. She prepared for likely eventualities as she shifted reporting relationships, and as her organization got ready for a new CEO and health care reform. She developed plans for the loss of her job, and she rehearsed important meetings. Equally significant, she became clear that her ultimate goal while in this position was to continue to be a respected member of the team, even if her own function was threatened.

In the end, LuAnn's history of excellence and these five strategies served her well. The new CEO arrived and, soon enough, her department and her position were eliminated. Throughout the process, LuAnn held her own. Others in the organization saw her as a valuable contributor even in the most onerous personal circumstances.

LuAnn was asked to stay in the organization. She now enjoys a new job that she helped to create and she still earns a competitive salary. She fuels her passion and uses her expertise every day, and she reports that she could not be happier with how she managed the process and the results she created for herself.

Yes, the individual who occupies the role of our boss certainly does matter, whether the new boss is the same as the old or not. But the individual who is reporting to the boss matters even more. LuAnn illustrates what can happen if we face our fears and we are honest about how real they are. When we practice being our best and plan for the worst, we can survive and prosper, regardless of what outside forces have in store.

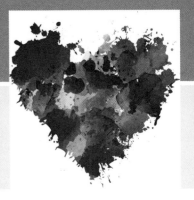

39

Know When to Go

Is it time for you to leave your job? How do you know when it's time to go? What are the cues that should alert you? What are the warning signals that you ignore to your detriment? This is the first of three chapters that investigate job changes—real and potential—when new circumstances unfold.

Over time, I have received many questions from readers, and as I was reviewing them, I was struck by a common theme: How do we know when it's time to move on?

What a great question. How many of us know leaders who have stayed too long on the job? When you think about those leaders, past or present, what stands out for you? Are they engaging, positive, and solicitous of feedback and ideas other than their own? Do they inspire you, and do you enjoy being around them?

Most likely your answers to those questions are no. So you know how it looks and feels when someone else has stayed too long, but how do you know about yourself?

HAVE YOU STAYED TOO LONG?

First, here are some signs and symptoms that should alert you about to own behavior and feelings.
- You no longer feel congruence between your job and who you really are. Your values and ethics are out of sync with those of your organization or your boss.
- Your dissatisfaction with your job is negatively affecting the rest of your life.
- You feel overloaded and burned out.
- You are more emotional than usual. You cry more often, either on or off the job, or both. You are also angry more often, either on or off the job, or both.
- You are working with people you no longer enjoy or respect.
- You are not learning from your boss.
- You have less energy than at other times in your life. You believe your health may be at risk, or you simply don't want to go to work.

Even if you are still emotionally engaged with your job, what are some signals from the outside that it's time to dust off your résumé?
- You are no longer invited to meetings and decision-making conversations that used to be routine for you.
- Your boss is not listening to or respecting your point of view.
- Your organization, unit, department, or service is no longer sustainable.
- Your organization or department is undergoing so much belt-tightening that your function may be on the line.
- Your coworkers or boss are acting differently toward you. They are more distant and their remarks are more circumspect than they have been in the past.

ASSESS THE SIGNALS

Both lists are filled with cues that warrant your attention. However, by themselves, none of these is a sure-fire reason to leave your job. Instead, they are warning signs that call for reflection about whether it's time for you to move on. Here's how you can tell if it is:

1. Think carefully about whether you still love what you do and where and how you do it *in this job*. If you were to make a ledger sheet with the pros and cons of this job, what would you put in each column? Do this exercise. What do the completed lists tell you? How long is each list? What weight do you give the entries in each column? For example, if you depend upon your paychecks for your livelihood, how important is it that *this job* provides your income? How likely is it that you will find an equivalent job or better, and what will it cost to obtain such a position? Is it worth it?

2. Assess what can and cannot be altered on your job, either by you or someone else. Assess whether you have done everything in your power to change troubling dynamics that are within your sphere of influence. Be scrupulously honest in your assessment. If you have not

acted on your own behalf, why haven't you? Sometimes we are truly powerless to change our circumstances, but many times we are not. Sometimes we are seduced by being needed on the job, even if we are needed too much. Sometimes we get stuck in our own "isn't it awful" story. Sometimes we render ourselves helpless when we are not. Sometimes we are convinced of everyone else's faults without considering our own contributions to our problems.

3. For factors that are outside your control, assess whether they can change, whether they will change, and if so, when change will occur. Consider whether you can live with what is likely to happen and when.

4. If you are experiencing unsatisfactory relationships with your coworkers or boss, assess whether these relationships can be repaired. Consider what part of these poor relationships you created yourself. Ask for input from trusted, knowledgeable others if you are not sure that your conclusions are correct.

If you determine that you can and should take action and address what's wrong, plan carefully and do not lead with your emotions. Or, if your list of pros and cons reveals that the best course of action is to stay put, do your best while you are still in your job. Readjust your thoughts and feelings by taking care of yourself and focusing on the pro side of your list. What do you genuinely appreciate about your job? What can you add to your list of pros? Post your list where you can see it and review it regularly.

If, however, you determine that your significant work relationships are damaged beyond repair, your job dissatisfiers are too great and not likely to shift soon enough, or you cannot exert sufficient influence to instigate the change you desire, it is time to move on.

If it is that time, know that you are in good company if you feel anxious about looking for another position, even if you are well qualified. Move ahead anyway. As Eunice Azzani[a] notes, "If work does not feed you and ignite your soul, it's time to rethink what you're doing. If you can't bring yourself to go to work, don't bring someone else."

YOU'RE LEAVING. NOW WHAT?

Let's say you've made the decision to leave. In addition to the obvious steps involved in looking for another job, as a masterful leader, what else do you do?

1. *Take control.* Create your departure plan. Work hard in your present position until the end. Take thoughtful action that respects your relationships with your coworkers, patients, and organization.

2. *Consider the legacy you want to leave.* Think about how you want to be remembered on this job. Think about what you will see when you look back. What will it take for you to feel good about the way in which you leave?

3. *Don't burn bridges.* Although health care consumes a staggeringly large proportion of our national expenditures each year, our community is surprisingly small. It is likely we will meet each other many times throughout our careers.

Remember that your career is yours to manage. Never forget that you have worked hard to earn your place at this table and the next one too.

---

[a]Azzani E. How to Leave a Job with Class Once You Know It's Over. http://wf.wetfeet.com/Experienced-Hire/On-the-job/Articles/How-to-Leave-a-Job-with-Class-Once-You-Know-It's-O.aspx. Accessed July 9, 2010.

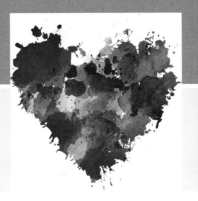

40

Managing an Exit

You plan to leave your job and you've been thought-ful about how and when to announce it. You've taken your manager's needs into account, as well as your own. But you're distressed when you receive unex-pected, unpleasant reactions to your news. How can you handle your disappointment with grace? What can you do to move on with your self-regard and dignity intact?

This is a story about Bonnie, a reader who generously offered her experience as a follow-up to the previous chap-ter (39), "Know When to Go." Bonnie's story is disguised to protect her identity, and we both hope that her experi-ence will benefit readers who leave their positions of their own accord.

Bonnie is a nurse leader who excelled in her institution and in her role for many years. She brought resources to her department, and she received recognition for her pro-fessional contributions to the field and for the achieve-ments she and her team accomplished. Not long ago, she began to seriously consider her future. After much thought and conversation with her family, she decided that it was time to leave her job. She did not wish to depart the orga-nization altogether, but she did want to make a change that would free her from the time commitments of her position.

Bonnie gave a lot of thought to what would best prepare the organization for her eventual change. She reasoned that telling her boss well ahead of her departure would allow for an orderly transition, so she decided to give 9 months' notice.

Much to her surprise, Bonnie's job changed dramati-cally within minutes of stating her intention to leave. Her boss asked several questions as Bonnie discussed her deci-sion to go, and by the time their meeting came to an end, her responsibilities had been greatly reduced. Bonnie left the meeting feeling she had no say in the changes; in fact, she felt devastated. Her boss's reaction not only surprised her, but it also left her feeling devalued and dismissed.

No matter what we think about Bonnie's timing and the reaction of her supervisor, her story provides a window into a somewhat common scenario. Although many health care organizations publicly honor the accomplishments of their leaders when they depart, events behind closed doors may not always be so positive. Unfortunately, Bonnie's experience vividly illustrates that we may need to prepare for a potentially abrupt transition when we decide it's time to leave.

Those who hold the leadership and managerial reigns in health care must ensure that the institution does its work in the highest-quality, most efficient, and cost-effective man-ner. They are there to ensure that the "trains run on time." When a leader or manager opts out of the place she occu-pies in the system, she sends a signal that the job for which she has been responsible must now be managed differently. No matter how deftly (or poorly) a supervisor handles this information, the leader needs to understand that the boss is going to move ahead as he or she sees fit.

Here are the things to consider when you decide to exit:

- *No matter how your colleagues respond to your deci-sion, don't take it personally,* especially if their reac-tions are disappointing. Some organizations are very skilled at honoring people and what "was," whereas others are not. Even when organizations excel at recog-nition, this truism still applies: nature abhors a vacuum. When we vacate our positions, the job needs to be filled. The well-being of the function and its domain becomes the focus of others' attention.
- *Along with that change in focus come new consider-ations and sometimes a heavy dose of politics as well.* This reality may take us by surprise. Worse, we may not agree with the directions that others decide to take. Although we can make a case for a different course of action, in the end we have signaled that we have let go of the reins. When we do that, our voices may be weakened.
- *Plan for different reactions.* Although the organization may sincerely praise you when you resign, be clear-headed about the possibility that your well-deserved acknowledgment may not be forthcoming in the way

you would like. You will be well served to expect different responses to your news because factors beyond your awareness may come into play immediately. Even if you don't anticipate exactly what happens, you will have thought through possibilities other than the best-case reply.

- *Buy time.* If you find yourself in the "give-notice" meeting like Bonnie did and your job is shifted immediately, say you want to sleep on it before you agree to changes that require your consent.
- *Think carefully about how much notice you provide your employer.* There is no single right answer to this critical question because the answer really does depend on several factors. However, there is one rule of thumb: if you think you need to provide a long lead time, consider cutting that time by at least half. Not all organizations will respond to such a lengthy transition as Bonnie's did, but some will. Bonnie found herself having her responsibilities parceled out within minutes of her announcement. Perhaps her boss's zeal is unusual, but the organization's need to adjust to the change is not.
- *Even if things go as planned, realize that as a leader who makes a big investment in your work, you may experience leaving that work as a significant loss.* Even when our reasons for making a job change are entirely positive and on our own terms, we may still feel the emotional sting of loss. When that happens, we need to be kind to ourselves, understand that these feelings are normal, and give ourselves as much self-care as possible.
- *Before you talk with your boss about your intention, be clear about what you want as you leave.* Don't assume that your boss and your organization will know what is best for you. It is up to you to initiate and negotiate the terms of your departure. How will your decision be communicated? Do you want a package? What responsibilities would you like to carry out before you leave?

What about training others; is that a role you want and is that a role the organization wants you to perform?

- *Once you have informed your supervisor that you are going, think carefully about what you are going to say to your peers, direct reports, etc.* Remember that in the absence of information, people will still find out you are leaving. In the absence of information you provide or authorize, people will make meaning of your exit anyway. It is human nature: when coworkers don't have *the* story, they will make up *a* story.
- *Before you resign, identify who is going to be your confidant during the process.* Select someone with whom you can candidly talk and who will support you no matter what. Is that a spouse, best friend, relative, or community member? When making your choice, be wary of selecting someone from the organization. Even if you are best friends with this individual, politics and split loyalties could change the dialogue and your relationship down the line.
- *Particularly when a departure is well into the future, realize that your power may diminish before you go.* This can be very difficult to experience and even more difficult to accept. It may help to remember that you initiated this change, and ultimately only you control how you will experience it. Even if you become less powerful in your role, you are still powerful as an individual and in the rest of your life. Lean into your own strength, your accomplishments, and the support of others so that you can stay confident, no matter what.

As Bonnie thought about her lessons learned, she realized that she had "temporary custody" rather than permanent guardianship over her function. She discovered that it never really was "her" job, even though she loved and embraced the work completely. For many years, she "owned" her role as fully as possible, but that ownership could not last forever. Neither could her tenure.

41

You've Left Your Job and the Unexpected Happens

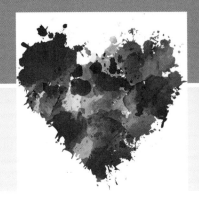

You have left your job, and much to your surprise, you are having real difficulty finding a new one. Why? What can you learn from your experience of seeking but not finding new work? How can you manage the stress, disappointment, and self-doubt you are experiencing? What can you do to refresh yourself so that you can compete successfully for a new role?

Most of us will change positions or relocate, or both, sometime during our careers. How are we going to handle these changes? What if a change is not one that we anticipate or initiate? How will that affect our emotions and our capacity to be our best when we interview? Will we demonstrate our excellence as leaders, or will we inadvertently convey negativity?

This chapter is dedicated to a reader who wanted to share her story of a job change. We will call her Pearl; we both hope that this anonymous tale of her circumstances will be valuable to you.

Pearl is an articulate, well-prepared nurse executive. She has held several positions as a chief nursing officer (CNO); a few years ago, she and her family moved to an unfamiliar part of the country to accommodate her husband's transfer. Pearl found a nurse executive position with relative ease, but after a few years her family missed their relatives and friends back home. They wanted to move back but had no definite time-line when Pearl began to search for a new position. At the same time, Pearl's organization began to establish new affiliations that affected her span of control. Eventually, Pearl's organization eliminated her position.

Soon after, her husband lost his job. Pearl's leisurely exploration for "just the right job" became a focused quest for a "good enough" position. After several CNO interviews didn't pan out, Pearl broadened her search to include nurse manager and service line positions.

We meet Pearl now that she has relocated. She's back in the comfort of home and family, but she's spent many months looking for a new job without success.

My time with Pearl has assured me that she is well-spoken and passionate about being a nurse leader. She has a vision for patient care and has experience that any organization would value. She is willing to sustain daily travel if her new job requires a commute. So, what is preventing Pearl from finding a new position? Here are some possibilities:

- In response to my questions, Pearl was eager to tell me a lot about her experience. She shared many details; she elaborated on how qualified she was and how many candidates there are for CNO positions. She talked about the long delays between recruiter and organizational responses to her interviews and phone calls. I wanted to hear these details, but if I were not a *very* interested party, I would probably stop listening when I became saturated with too much information. What if interviewers and recruiters had the same reaction? When we are in Pearl's situation, it is natural to tell our stories in full. But we have to discern which audience wants to hear the unabridged version. Recruiters and chief executive officers are not receptive to too many details when they are unrelated to their questions.
- Pearl broadened her search to include nurse manager and service line roles, and after extensive interviews and lengthy delays, she was told repeatedly that she was overqualified. Going forward, Pearl will get more information before investing time and emotional "capital" in jobs she has little chance to land.
- Pearl will work to increase her self-awareness. What's difficult at this point in a lengthy search is that our emotions become frayed, and we can become tired, upset, and frustrated. These are understandable reactions, but if we aren't managing them, they can corrode our capacities to interview well.

MANAGING A PROTRACTED JOB SEARCH

What else can Pearl do as she continues her search?

- *Lead with her strong suit.* There is no doubt that Pearl is a passionate nurse leader. But the clarity of her commitment didn't come out until long after I'd heard lots of stories. Most of these stories were about unsuccessful results, lengthy delays in response, poor outcomes from interviews, and frustration with the process. It took a long time for Pearl to reveal the true passion, expertise, and vision that she can offer any organization.
- *Take care of herself.* Getting enough sleep, eating right, exercising, networking, and keeping current in the profession are all important activities during any job search. But they are especially important in a lengthy search where there is so much pressure to be successful.
- *Be around supportive people.* Pearl can be deliberate about where she turns for the emotional support she needs and deserves. She needs to have people with whom she can share her stories and frustrations. She also needs to have regular contact with people who will comfort her and remind her of her value and excellence as a nurse leader.
- *Seek honest feedback.* Pearl can request feedback when an interview does not yield positive results. When she receives this feedback, she can "check the fit." Sometimes, feedback is way off, but there are times when it is spot on or contains at least a grain of truth.
- *Remember projection.* On occasion, people simply don't "like" us because something about us rubs them the wrong way. Maybe we look like a relative they don't enjoy. When we are highly qualified but not selected, it's possible that this is an (unstated and unconscious) reason.
- *Have a candid colleague in her corner.* Pearl can seek the counsel of people who will challenge her from time to time. Although supportive people are a must, so are people who see and respect us but who think differently than we do.
- *Watch her stories.* Pearl has had a challenging struggle, and we have already looked at the results of sharing too much of that struggle with others in professional settings. The stories Pearl tells herself can be equally damaging because they can depress her or worse. To balance the picture, Pearl can consider appreciative questions such as what she is grateful for. What has she learned that she can take forward? What "good" outcomes has this journey given Pearl?

Pearl is going to keep doing the footwork to secure a new job, and she is going to employ these and related strategies while she does it. She will stay lovingly engaged with people and projects she enjoys. Knowing Pearl, she will undoubtedly achieve her goal soon.

Claiming Your Power and Your Place

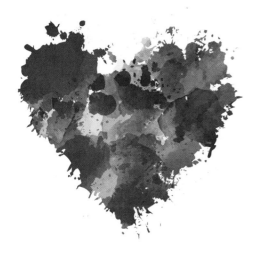

You are more powerful than you know. As you ripen, claim, and act on your influence, you can make an even bigger contribution to the world of health care and patient well-being. When you practice reflecting and learning, staying true to your values, navigating change, and managing your relationships so they thrive, you cannot help but become a more powerful leader.

This section is about owning your growth, claiming your voice, and becoming the masterful leader you were meant to be. It addresses how to confidently move into positions of greater authority, and how to deal with the powerful "detractors" that you may experience along the way.

42

You've Been an "Emerging Leader" Long Enough

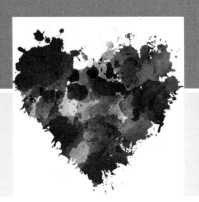

You are a relatively new leader. But you're clinically experienced and well groomed in the ways of leadership. Opportunities to take the reins abound. Are you ready? You know there is never a sure way of knowing, so you decide to "go for it." Here's how.

This chapter is about a dialogue I recently had with Antonia, a nurse leader who will turn 40 this year. Antonia shared that she has been honored to have several outstanding mentors who have provided her counsel and genuine friendship in recent years. One of those trusted mentors is retiring soon, and a number of Antonia's other colleagues are also taking leave of their senior leadership roles. So, now Antonia and other once-young leaders are moving into the positions previously occupied by mentors who were more seasoned and experienced.

This has given Antonia pause as she considers the doors that are opening around her. In a candid conversation, she shared her thoughts and feelings about the changes she sees and the challenges and opportunities she is experiencing.

With Antonia's permission, I offer a snapshot of our conversation. Although these views may be the same or different than yours, our hope is that the ideas here will stimulate reflection and dialogue. What are your thoughts about the "changing of the guard," the implications of that change, and the best ways forward for the next generation of nurse leaders?

Here are a few of Antonia's reactions to the eminent departure of her mentors:

1. On balance, Antonia feels well prepared for increasingly responsible leadership roles. She frequently acknowledges the generosity and wisdom of the mentors who have helped her gain this level of preparation.

2. Antonia also acknowledges that she did not always feel welcomed or "ready" for leadership. In fact, when she first became a manager, she felt that her voice was tolerated but not solicited. Fortunately, that changed over time, and Antonia attributes much of that change to the sensitivity of the leaders around her. They became aware of their own limiting biases about "emerging leaders," and when they did, they consciously opened their minds and encouraged broader participation at the leadership table.

3. Despite her growth and supportive colleagues, Antonia still feels a bit intimidated when she works with "leadership experts." Antonia has opinions, and she believes they are valid, but she often holds back while more seasoned others speak their minds. As she told me this, it was clear that Antonia has compassion for herself. She is not "beating herself up," but even so, she has two concerns about her reluctance to speak up:
   a. Without arrogance, she wonders whether her reticence causes her to withhold information that could lead to better decisions, and
   b. What will she and others like her do when the senior leaders are no longer there?

IT'S YOUR TURN

Antonia's last question paved the way for the rest of our conversation. As a generation of leaders retires, what insights and reflective questions might be helpful for younger leaders whose peers and mentors are departing? Here are a few of our thoughts:

1. ***When your leadership is called for, do not sit it out and wait until you are asked to step up.*** Instead, pause and give the situation your undivided and thoughtful

attention, even if it is just for a few minutes. Then take your best shot. If it helps, think about what your mentor or another admired leader would do in the same situation.

2. ***Watch others as they lead and consider what works and what does not.*** This is common advice, yet its importance cannot be overstated. It is easy to forget to observe behavior and impact when we are busy meeting the demands on us every day.

3. ***Do the right thing as you understand it at the time.*** Then reflect and learn from your successes and mistakes.

4. ***Ask trusted others for their feedback when you are not certain about how you are doing.*** Then consider the "fit" of the feedback. Does it ring true? Is the feedback about you and your leadership in the situation, or is it mostly a projection of the provider's personality and wishes? Both types of feedback are common; either way, what portion of the feedback is useful to your own learning and growth?

5. ***Frame your feedback requests clearly so your colleagues can give you specific rather than general information.*** If you do not get what you need with your initial question, don't hesitate to ask for clarification. For example,

"Can you tell me how I sounded when I led that meeting?" could lead to a flattering but not particularly helpful answer like "you were great." If that happens, you can ask for more precise feedback by saying "Thank you. In what ways did my approach work for you?" That could lead to an answer with more details: "You spoke unemotionally, and your requests were logical and easy to understand."

6. ***If you have the opportunity, talk with your departing mentors about how you are feeling before they go.*** If you are inclined, ask them about how they are feeling too. Let them know that their work and influence will not end when they leave because they have instilled them in you. Let them know what you are excited about, and what causes you some concern, intimidation, or fear. Invite their suggestions for how to move forward.

7. ***As new opportunities come your way, notice how you feel and reflect on when you have felt this way before.*** What was the situation, and what feelings did you have? How did you move through your feelings and the challenges you faced? What worked well and what was not so successful? What does your past experience teach you about what to do now?

43

Demonstrate Courage and Own Your Power

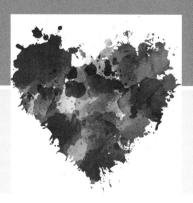

Many of us have career-constricting habits such as needing to be needed and having to be right. However, with practice and self-care, you can let go of these and other professionally limiting behaviors. This is courageous work, and when you engage in it, you will be well positioned to step into and embrace your personal power. Here are the ways to do it.

Judi is a nurse who performs reasonably well in her job as a hospital manager. Her position doesn't come with a big budget, but she knows how to work cooperatively with people to achieve her goals and the goals they share together. She is hard working and generally acknowledged for doing her work well enough.

But for some time now, Judi has known that she is not as effective as she could be. When she is honest with herself, she recognizes that she often acts in unproductive ways. Although she may look good on the surface, like a duck appearing to glide easily on smooth water, Judi is paddling very hard underneath.

Judi knows that some of her habits limit her potential for success, not only at work but also in the rest of her life. So, recently, she developed a kind of inventory of her unproductive behaviors. She did this because she wanted to identify and understand more about her actions and motivations. Here is a short list of the unproductive behavior patterns she identified:

- Judi has a hard time saying no. She takes on too much and then tries to do it all, discounting the personal or professional cost. She works long hours, and consequently, her relationships suffer. She is tired almost all of the time, and there are warning signs that her physical health is affected by her lack of exercise, poor nutrition, and insufficient rest.
- Related to her reluctance to say no, Judi recognizes that she wants to be needed. When colleagues ask for her help, she feels validated and wanted. She doesn't like to admit it, but she says she seeks the appreciation

that others offer when she says yes. Her strong need for gratefulness has been unconscious until now, but at this point, Judi sees that this robust drive has preempted other imperatives such as taking better care of herself.
- Judi has a hard time setting and sticking to priorities. Like many health care managers, her job is complex, and there are frequent day-to-day "fires" that capture her attention, even when they are not urgent. Judi has sought out new tools and training in time management, but after these events, she admits that she hasn't reviewed her learning or practiced new time-saving techniques.
- Judi has a strong distaste for conflict. For example, she is quite bothered when direct reports don't perform as they should. But when she has the chance to coach or teach them to do better, she shies away if doing so will require a tough conversation. Instead, when direct reports are not pulling their weight, she goes out of her way to be "nice" and gives them second and third chances. She tells herself that she does this because she wants to be supportive, and she believes this is true, in part. But the rest of the story is that she doesn't want to confront or set boundaries because it will make her feel uncomfortable.

As Judi reflected on these and other ineffective patterns, she realized that she often takes the easy way out of difficult situations. Saying "yes" too much, avoiding conflict, and succumbing to being needed and appreciated are ways of "self-soothing" or opting to feel good in the moment. There is nothing wrong with feeling good, but when it is done at the expense of taking initiative and doing the right thing, it is self-defeating. Eventually, we can become blind to the big price we are paying for our unwillingness to challenge ourselves to grow and excel.

So what is that big price? Maybe we will feel a little badly that we've taken the easy road, but there is a much bigger and more damaging consequence—the loss of our personal power as a leader. Being exhausted, not attending to staff performance issues, and sacrificing long-term priorities for short-term "emergencies" all take a toll on our effectiveness and our value in the eyes of others. When we have sacrificed best practice for what is easiest, we have diminished our power, authority, and leadership potential.

We may not realize it, but by succumbing to and gratifying our immediate needs versus tending to the more important responsibilities of our roles, we have reduced our capacity to think about and to choose *how we want to be* as a leader. Do we want to be effective by making thoughtful decisions, opting for difficult choices when needed, and engaging in challenging conversations? Or do we want to self-soothe and lose the opportunity to do right by our leadership positions, our patients, and the people we want to influence?

SMALL STEPS CAN BE COURAGEOUS

Judi decided to stop being hijacked by her short-term emotional needs. Instead, she vowed to be more courageous and practice being the leader she knew she could be, even if it caused her some initial discomfort. Here is what she chose to do when she was tempted to take the easy way out:

1. ***Count to 10 and breathe deeply while doing it.*** This simple act prompts a biological reset; we feel more relaxed, and we are better able to think about our options versus reacting in the moment. Doing this is a healthful way to buy time.

2. ***After breathing deeply, Judi decided she wouldn't address the issue until she'd had a chance to make a considered decision about what to do.*** She wanted to reflect, even if just for a moment, on the problem. If she needed to respond immediately, she would say something like "please give me a minute." This would allow her to mentally step out of the situation and observe it as a third party might see it. Observing, even for a moment, would provide her with a fresh perspective on the circumstances as well as the other players and herself.

3. ***When a courageous action was called for, Judi pledged that she would not make excuses or hide.*** She dedicated herself to rehearsing tough conversations before they happened when she had that luxury, and she also promised herself that she would practice saying "give me a minute" and "no." She knew she might be clumsy with these words at first, so she also gave herself permission to keep trying until they came naturally.

Finally, Judi vowed to refresh her vision and purpose as a leader. She was genuinely dedicated to good patient care and her role in providing it. She also believed in personal humility and service. Judi knew that if she stayed focused on her values and potential, she would find the courage to practice, grow, and eventually excel in her leadership role.

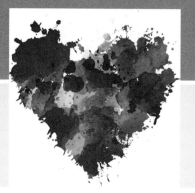

44

How Do You See Yourself?

Is your view of yourself as a leader aligned with how others see you? How can you check your story about yourself? One way is to ask trusted others for feedback. Make it safe for them to be honest, and then reflect carefully on what they say. Those who lead with heart and mastery are not shy about getting input to enhance their self-knowledge, congruence, and effectiveness.

How aligned are your intentions and outcomes? How comparable are your images of yourself with the ways others see you?

Why do I invite you to consider these questions? Often leadership coaching involves exploration of these questions. Each of us carries filters, distortions, and other impediments that prevent us from being honest with ourselves. An unintentional lack of truthfulness about how we portray ourselves can seriously limit our efficacy with others.

Nurse leaders who take the time to get real about who they are, what they think, how they feel, and what they truly value have a clear picture of themselves as leaders. When they couple these reflective questions with queries about their impact on others, they have a far better chance of being congruent with themselves and others. They also have a far better chance of achieving the results they desire.

Here we address just one aspect of leading with this type of congruence—leadership presence. In this chapter, leadership presence means correspondence between our beliefs about ourselves and the way we actually appear to others. How accurate is the story we tell ourselves about our effectiveness? What blind spots might we have about our real impact on others? How similar are our words compared with the nonverbal messages we send? Do we present a coherent picture? Since we are the leadership "vehicle" for our message, is that vehicle harmonious or discordant?

Here is a true story about my coaching client, Olga. She has held a leadership role in a complex health system for several years, and she has earned multiple degrees, secured elected positions, and received accolades throughout her career.

Recently, she asked me to accompany her to an event in which she was an observer. While we were there, she was asked to speak spontaneously to a large group of her nurse leader colleagues. She arose, spoke for a few minutes, and returned to her seat.

Later, we reviewed what she had done with this unexpected opportunity to address the group. When she asked for my assessment, I said I thought she was articulate, powerful in her delivery, and just a little bit stiff. I asked what she thought of her public moment. She said she perceived herself to be tongue-tied and awkward, with nothing to say. In fact, she was embarrassed about how she had shown up in the group.

Our versions of what had occurred were quite different. We discussed further and realized that Olga frequently sees herself as being ineffective in group settings. I have seen her in many such circumstances, and I let her know that I see her impact as significant and powerful. As her trusted advisor, I was not saying this to assuage Olga. Nor do I believe my truth is necessarily "the" truth. But, with my view, Olga had another perspective to consider.

If Olga had not sought another opinion, what might the consequence have been? First, she would be living within the confines of her unchecked story. Given her belief that she had embarrassed herself, it is possible that Olga would have been demure in conversations after the meeting. It's possible that her post-meeting demeanor would diminish her power and potential in the eyes of others.

To be sure, her colleagues' prior experience would inform their views of Olga prior to this incident. Still, it's quite possible that Olga's belief about the event and her likely self-deprecating actions afterward could create a self-fulfilling prophecy: others could perceive her as awkward and not very powerful.

Longer-term consequences might be even more significant. Because I work with Olga, I know that she has limited herself to roles that are satisfactory but not challenging. I know that she has hesitated to pursue her big professional dream. I know that she has procrastinated on tasks that will help her actualize the contribution she really wants to make to nursing and health care. She is not playing the bigger game that she is entirely capable of playing.

This is just one example of a leader's interaction among thousands of others. While you and I cannot stop the action to reflect on the subtleties of every exchange, look at the value Olga received by asking about just one moment of her day.

ASKING FOR EXTERNAL FEEDBACK

As you think about whether and how this story applies to you, ask yourself whether you want outside input to assess the accuracy and impact of the leadership picture you are presenting. If you do, here are several tools you can use.

Solicit the input of others. 360° instruments provide important information about how we are perceived by others. Less formal feedback can be equally valuable. In this instance, Olga asked for my impression after a few moments of speaking with a group. Had she not sought another's point of view, she would have lived within only her own self-diminishing story about the event.

Make it safe for others to respond. For people to respond openly, they need to feel respected, valued, and protected. They need to know their honesty will not cause retribution.

Consider the questions you want to ask. Some examples are: "What did you notice about me in that situation?" "What did you experience as a positive?" "What was not so positive or otherwise distracting for you?" "What impact do you think I had?"

Thank those who respond. Knowing that you have received the message well, regardless of its content, will support and deepen your relationship with this person. It will also create the conditions for you to receive more helpful feedback in the future.

Realize the limitations of others' points of view. The comments of others are offered through the lens of their own perspectives. This is true for all of us, regardless of our intentions. It is always possible that the input says more about the sender than it says about you.

Check the fit. Feedback offers us new information. It is our responsibility to consider whether and how accurate the data are for us. You can ask yourself whether this perspective is valid for you. Is any part of it valid? If so, what might you be doing to create these impressions? What other curiosities do you have?

Consider your follow-up. Do you want to change an observation that concerns you? Do you want to take any action? If you believe that making a shift has merit, yet you are resisting, what is your resistance about?

Determine if you want or need support as you make this change. If you decide to take action, do you need support? If so, what mechanisms or agreements do you need to put in place?

The benefits of leading with congruence and alignment are considerable. In this example, Olga later added this feedback to other input that was equally positive. As a result, she has learned about her impact on others. She reports feeling more confident. She is more self-assured and satisfied, and she is moving forward toward her dream with greater momentum. This simple exercise helped to remove a real barrier for Olga.

Leaders whose presence sends congruent messages are more likely to be perceived credibly. Close alignment of your words, your overall presence, and your stated values are powerful. Congruence and alignment allow others to listen to your messages more fully; they are not distracted by messages that simply don't track.

The greater your leadership congruence, the more likely you are to be heard with the full measure of your intent. I invite you to embrace the exciting and rewarding journey to owning the full measure of your power and effectiveness.

45

Being a One-Person Show

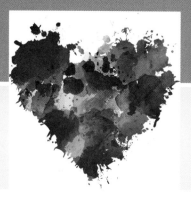

An aspiring nurse leader is challenged by her need to be a "one-person" show. She wants to overcome this because she knows that thriving leaders share power and willingly collaborate with other leaders. Masterful leaders don't have to be the only leadership voice in the room. If the need to be a "one-person show" applies to you at times, here are ways to overcome your ego's wishes to take center stage too often.

Nurse leaders never fail to inspire me. In this chapter, I want to honor Allison, a young leader who is new to her role as a chief nursing officer (CNO). Allison describes herself as fully committed to patient care and leadership excellence. She is committed to understanding and learning from her mistakes, and she is eager to express her power differently. Her story offers all of us lessons in being flexible in service of leading with the best of our skills and intentions.

When she began in her new role as CNO a year ago, Allison was convinced she could do a great job, and she was determined to show that from the start. She was committed to letting her new colleagues know that she is a strong, decisive, and capable leader. She fulfilled this intention by leading from "in front" in nearly every encounter. Instead of showing interest in her coworkers by asking for their thoughts when the situation called for it, she shared her own opinions first. Then she took action, frequently without the benefit of anyone else's input.

As her first-year anniversary approached, Allison elected to work with a coach because she sensed that her choice to lead with forceful conviction was not being well received. As it turned out, her first-year review and a subsequent 360° process confirmed that her peers, boss, and subordinates had serious concerns about Allison's fit with the organization.

The good news for Allison was that all of her coworkers acknowledged her competence, and they appreciated her values and command of nursing and patient safety matters.

However, they had other serious worries. Their negative feedback centered on Allison's approach to relationships and the way she treated those around her. They felt that she did not show respect for others' longevity. She also did not exhibit interest in their opinions, even when they were the experts and more familiar with the context than Allison. Furthermore, several of her colleagues said she was arrogant, excessively pushy, and overly focused on herself. They also stated that she was easily rattled when challenged; they described her as lacking the ability to converse and reflect. They believed she was "shooting from the hip" on many occasions.

Allison saw it differently. When a subordinate or a peer asked many questions or wanted more information about her direction, Allison believed that these were efforts to undermine her leadership. She felt that her peers or direct reports were being insubordinate and disrespectful when they didn't immediately go along with her decisions.

Allison's reaction to her experience of insubordination was to double down—she became even more forceful. By her own account, she struck back "reflexively," sometimes blurting out that a decision had been made or that a questioning colleague was simply wrong. She explained to me that her motivation was to display more power and more knowledge than her "opponent."

For her colleagues, the consequences of Allison's reactions were troublesome at best and gravely concerning at worst. Her boss and peers knew that Allison was intent on staying in her job, but they were not so sure. One reason was that they were committed to multidisciplinary collaboration, and they felt Allison's behavior was egotistical and her viewpoint was too "nursing-centric." Further, their experience of Allison's "decisive" leadership was that it created resistance and even animosity among her equally talented peers and direct reports.

So, how did Allison turn this around?

1. *She reflected on what was causing her to communicate that she was better and smarter than those around her.* She understood that expressing her power by dominating was bound to be a turn-off to the very people upon whom her success depended.

2. *She got clarity on her long-term vision of success, and she identified the intersections between her vision with that of the organization and the rest of the leadership team.* Based on their common goals, she articulated what she wanted to achieve and how she wanted to relate to her colleagues.

3. *She saw the limits of leading with solely her own knowledge.* She realized that intelligence, experience, and decisiveness were not enough to nurture strong relationships with her colleagues.

4. *She recognized the corrosive power of her bad habits.* She saw that being unwavering in nearly every situation was back-firing. If she couldn't temper ill-serving behaviors such as speaking first and lacking curiosity about other people and their perspectives, she could wind up losing her job.

5. *She considered how she sounded when disagreeing with a colleague or direct report.* She thought about how often she was communicating—essentially— that she was right and the other person was wrong.

6. *She reminded herself that her direct reports never forget that her role is more powerful than theirs.* She also took solace in knowing that her boss and peers believe she is competent. She saw that there was no need to restate or overstate her power and competence with any of her coworkers.

7. *She practiced interrupting her reflexive habits.*
   a. She focused on breathing before speaking or responding.
   b. She paid attention to being patient and waiting at least a day before she responded to irritating emails.
   c. She tried being curious and asking others how she could best support them rather than making demands that others support her.

8. *Finally, Allison had the courage to share her behavior change strategy with her colleagues, inviting their feedback and support as she moved forward.*

Now Allison is ready to demonstrate respect for her coworkers and work toward collaborative solutions rather than one-way pronouncements. It has not been easy, and Allison says she is still a work in progress. But she is starting to reap the benefits of her commitment to change. She knows that it will take time to foster productive and enjoyable relationships. Still, she has impressed us all with her ability to adapt to new ways of working together. She shows no sign of bitterness or resentment; in fact, she seems happier and truly eager to work from a position of power that honors others as well as herself.

46

The Power of Executive Presence

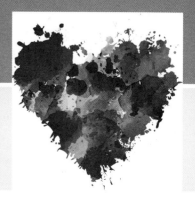

Executive presence is at once an attainable skill and a way of being. Here, we explore the importance of executive presence in nurse leaders, as confirmed by the American Organization for Nursing Leadership's Nurse Executive Competencies.[1a] We also review what executive presence means for you, and how you can develop and increase your own unique expression of it.

I have the privilege of working with some of health care's finest and most effective nursing leaders and their teams. Whether they are at the helm of large organizations or serving as managers with smaller spheres of influence, these individuals embody an intangible characteristic that signals strength, dignity, direction, and focus.

In my 2013 book, *Leading Valiantly in Healthcare*,[b] I call this quality "valor," and its manifestation is always unique. Other appropriate terms are "courageous," "inspiring," and "visionary." Regardless of which words appeal to you, what is important about all of them is that they convey a leader's own version of "executive presence."

What does it mean to possess executive presence? The word "presence" is ubiquitous in current leadership literature because it is profoundly important. Managers and leaders with executive presence have the skill to stay grounded, express authority, and lead powerfully on a regular basis. At the same time, they remain true to themselves. They are comfortable in their own skin, and even when they receive information that ruffles them, they know what to do to regain their composure.

Yet, leaders with "executive presence" are more than just authentic and grounded. They also "know their hearts"; that is, they have the capacity to stand by their agenda and relate to the rest of us. These leaders are not distracted. Instead, they hold to their beliefs as they remain in the dialogue that is their work. They do this through corporate highs and lows. They do it through professional relationship highs and lows too, whether those relationships are one on one, inside a team, or in a larger organizational setting.

Just how important is executive presence? In my experience, executive presence is a requisite skill and "way of being" for the health care and nurse managers who are most effective in guiding others, regardless of the specific environmental challenges they face. For another perspective, consider the American Organization of Nurse Executives' Nurse Executive Competencies.[c] These competencies are positioned as capabilities for managers at all levels; executive presence might be considered foundational for at least two of the five categories: communication/relationship building and leadership.

ENHANCING YOUR EXECUTIVE PRESENCE

Here are some ways to develop and increase your own executive presence:

1. ***Call to mind leaders who, in your opinion, possess executive presence.*** What qualities do they possess, and what is the impact of those qualities on you? Do you have these qualities? What is your impact on others? If you don't know the answers to these questions, ask for feedback from several people you trust.

2. ***Consider the effect of your body language.*** Notice whether you stand tall and straight, and how you position yourself when you speak with others. Observe

[a]AONL. Nurse Executive Competencies, 2011. http://www.aonl.org/resources/leadership%20tools/nursecomp.shtmi. Accessed April 18, 2014.

[b]Robinson-Walker, C. *Leading Valiantly in Healthcare: Four Steps to Sustainable Success*. Indianapolis, IN: Sigma Theta Tau International, Honor Society of Nursing; 2013.

[c]See footnote in the Introduction for the AONL Competencies.

whether your arms are routinely folded across your chest; this can suggest that you are not open to them or their input. Become conscious of how much eye contact you maintain. If your daily routine precludes you from observing your own body language, pay close attention to the reactions others have to you.

3. *Reduce distractions.* Most of us have too much on our plates, but leaders with executive presence manage the perception that they are too busy. They stay focused, and they want you to do the same thing. They too have many pulls on their time and attention, but they are able to compartmentalize. They don't become distracted by what's not relevant in a given task or conversation. When their attention is diverted for a few minutes, they readily return to their agenda.

4. *Develop self-awareness, understanding, and compassion for yourself.* How often do you notice how you are feeling emotionally and physically? When you do, do you take a few minutes for self-care when it can improve the way you are leading and communicating?

5. *Notice how you are relating to others.* Are you asking more than telling? Are you connecting with your colleagues authentically and with an approach that will enhance your relationships and your outcomes? Are you appreciating their efforts, and listening to understand versus to judge?

6. *Consider how much confidence you convey.* If you are a newer manager or leader and could use more confidence, are you accessing the resources that will help you develop your skills and your unique executive presence? If you have accomplished a lot in your career or on your job, do you "own" these successes? Have you mined these and other experiences for the lessons they can teach you? Do you deflate or inflate the significance of your contributions when you are interacting with others?

7. *Unearth the learning from the parts of your journey that were not successful.* Leaders with executive presence learn from all their experiences, not just their successes. The authority they convey and the admiration they evoke are frequently inspired by both wisdom and humility.

8. *Know how to get your poise back.* As noted earlier, even leaders with the most composure lose it from time to time. To regain your executive presence, your most readily available resource is your breath. Breathing brings calmness and the capacity to redirect your attention to what is most important. In addition, if you have a vision for yourself as a truly effective leader, call it to mind. What adjustments can you make to help you achieve your vision?

9. *Practice.* If you want to strengthen or develop new behaviors that demonstrate your unique executive presence, try them out. You may want to experiment by walking with more confidence, pausing to think before you speak, making more eye contact, and adjusting your ratio of telling versus asking and listening. Practice these behaviors in "safe" settings at first, and keep at it if the shifts feel uncomfortable when you start. Elicit feedback on what's working from those you trust, and keep doing those things that send the message you want to convey.

Executive presence is a way of being that is worth cultivating. Indeed, it is a uniquely effective "signature" for nurse leaders and managers who can combine it with their clinical knowledge and leadership skill to inspire others and lead with clarity.

47

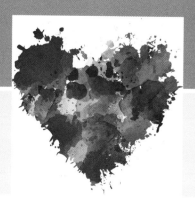

Leadership Blind Spots

How many of us have heard (or said), "that's just the way we do things here," even if these ways of doing business do not serve patients or staff? These are "blind spots," and we can all name examples of organizational allowances that are counter productive, but that are accepted anyway. Just one example is a poor performer whose manager does not address the problem or its negative effect on others. Masterful nurse leaders own their power by courageously addressing ill-serving behaviors such as letting poor performers just "get by."

Just exactly what is a blind spot? Technically, it is "an area in which one fails to exercise judgment or discrimination."[a] Leadership blind spots are significant aspects of institutional life in which we, the stewards of our organizations, fail to exercise our best judgment.

In fact, we may not even realize that we have a blind spot. Our bodies provide a good metaphor for understanding blind spots. As we know, unassisted human vision does not give us a 360-degree view of our surroundings. When we drive, we need rear- and side-view mirrors to access all the information we need to drive safely. Similarly, as leaders, it's not easy for us to see all of the organizational dynamics that affect our work, colleagues, and outcomes. To compensate, we need to gather other viewpoints. We must be intentional about seeking opinions and data so we can access the otherwise unknown factors that influence our efforts.

In this chapter we explore examples of organizational blind spots and dynamics that are both pernicious and destructive. I am referring to our unwitting acceptance of ineffective communication, inadequate managerial follow-through, and compromised support for new leaders.

Here are a few examples:

We place novices and advanced beginners in new leadership roles without providing them adequate formal learning and support. I have heard stories from countless nurse managers who are new to their positions but who have not received suitable training or proper assistance for their roles. We can do a much better job in this area. I teach a number of nurse leader and manager courses, and I hear many substantiating tales from those who attend. However, once they are exposed to appropriate learning programs, these new leaders are grateful beyond measure for the opportunities their supervisors have given them. They feel they finally have the chance to learn the competencies and skills they need. When their learning programs conclude, these beginner leaders leave with current knowledge and active support from new friends and colleagues. They show truly remarkable enthusiasm for their roles; in fact, they are downright eager to get back home so they can tackle the tough issues that face them.

Too frequently, we don't address poor attitudes and behavior in forthright ways. If we inherit individual performers with bad attitudes and unsuitable professional behavior, we demur or permit others to demur because we are conflict averse or "it was like this when I arrived." I hear many stories from managers who come into new jobs only to find individual performers who drag down the team. Sometimes these managers are caught in the middle: they know they should tackle the bad behavior, but the nurse in question

---

[a]Blind spot. Merriam-Webster Dictionary. Available at *www.merriam-webster.com.* Accessed May 2008.

has a longer tenure than the new manager. To make matters worse, their supervisors may not be available to help deal with the problem. Because these dynamics existed before they got there and because they don't have the skills or backing they need to challenge the longer-term nurse, the new managers default. They say the issues are simply too difficult to address. Or they turn a blind eye.

These new leaders are paying the price for the organization's long-standing, unintended "permission giving" for bad behavior. If individual performance issues were not dealt with in the past, then the organization unwittingly failed to carry out its responsibility. In comes the new manager. Without support, the new leader is in a difficult and unenviable spot. She may even be at risk for remaining in her new role. But with support, this new leader can learn from work with her supervisor. Together, they can develop a plan and appropriately address the problem.

We hear, we tell, and we unconsciously propagate institutional stories that are not helpful. How many of us have said or heard this statement: "That is just the way it is done around here"? While there are times when this is the right response, is it always the right response? How many of us have said those very same words without thinking about the message we are sending? In a time-tested leadership article called "Skilled Incompetence,"[b] Harvard professor Chris Argyris describes such categorical responses as "organizationally defensive routines." He defines these routines as, "(statements)…action(s) or polic(ies) designed to avoid surprise, embarrassment, or threat." "Organizationally defensive" statements like "that is just the way we do things" can become efficient ways to shut down legitimate questions and subtle challenges to the established order—even when such questions could lead to improving our processes and outcomes.

We send ambiguous messages. Unclear communication about roles, responsibilities, authority, and accountability will dilute the message and confuse the listener, even those with the best intentions. As communicators, we too have the best of intentions. But sometimes in our rush to manage our ever-growing responsibilities, we may take communication shortcuts that leave others perplexed. Sooner or later, our lack of clarity will cause a problem for these individuals, teams, the organization, or all of the above. The consequences could be costly in terms of muddied roles, poor accountability, and low morale. We must pay keen attention to the messages we send and seek feedback to ensure we are clear. Doing this will go a long way toward creating mutual understanding and cohesive action.

LEARNING FROM BLIND SPOTS

What lessons do these examples of leadership blind spots offer us? Our organizations will benefit when we:

1. *Encourage our colleagues, peers, and direct reports to give us feedback and ask questions.*
2. *Give permission for others to examine "sacred cows" or "the ways we have always done it."*
3. *Explore and address long-standing interpersonal problems.* Prepare for difficult conversations. Provide role-playing opportunities so leaders can practice and become more confident in dealing with challenging behaviors and attitudes. Be present in meetings where new supervisors need your active backing.
4. *Evaluate standing meetings and other routine activities.* Ask for ideas for better ways to accomplish routine tasks. Create a culture of openness and innovation.
5. *Ask employees, direct reports, and team members how you can support them so they can be more open with their thoughts and ideas.* This is especially helpful when you want to create a high-performance culture that is truly rich in feedback.
6. *Encourage people to say "I don't know" when they really don't know the answers.* Leaders who themselves say "I don't know" send the signal that it is okay to be less-than-expert in every area. When we do this, we model our own commitment to continuing our learning and displaying humility. With our words and actions, we are allowing others to do the same.

---

[b]Argyris C. Skilled incompetence. *Harvard Business Review.* September 1986.

48

If Only They Would Change

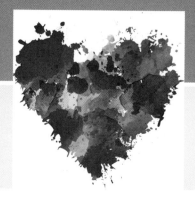

You observe that a senior-level executive doesn't understand a significant part of his job. You want to report this, and you know you are right and your colleague is wrong. But is that enough to carry the day? No, often it is not. We might know we are right, but in fact, being right and righteous about it is often a dead end. What can we do to focus less on others' flaws and more on managing our righteousness so we can be the influential leaders we want to be?

Sara is a young nurse leader with loads of potential. A few years ago, she left direct patient care to take an advocacy role in her local area, and last year, she took another advocacy position with a large association. She is eager to focus her considerable talents on health care policies that will make life better for patients and the institutions that serve them.

Sara is hard working, and she never shirks from fully preparing for the challenges before her. She also has a strong sense of right and wrong. While this usually serves her well, recently she began to feel frustrated with how things are versus how they "should be." She was especially irritated with several of the health care CEOs in her region. She said they didn't know the substance of key policy directives; she also complained that they talked down to her because she is young and attractive.

It is reasonable that Sara was concerned that her colleagues didn't know key elements of their jobs, and it is also understandable that she was distressed by what she considered to be poor professional behavior from people who were many years her senior. She was justified in expecting better.

But Sara couldn't let go of her indignation. She insisted that she was right to be incensed, and she complained that she was hindered by their bad behavior. She was quite emotional when she talked about her colleagues' transgressions and their effects on her. Unfortunately, some of her other peers started to complain about Sara's own "bad behavior."

They experienced her grievances as whining and immature, and they wanted her to "get over it and move on."

Sara's work relationships consequently began to suffer, and she started facing trouble focusing on important policy initiatives. She knew she was not at her best, but she couldn't see a way out of her predicament. She said she was stuck because she was right and the CEOs were wrong, and she didn't see that she could, or should, change herself when it was her older colleagues who should change.

Many of us can relate to Sara's dilemma because we too have been caught in the web of other people's imperfections and their effects on us. It can be quite difficult to see that other people's poor behavior can adversely affect how we behave too. It's also difficult to accept that other people don't always behave the way we think they should. We too may have asked what Sara was asking: How can I maintain my high standards and continue to work productively when those who should know better fall short of my expectations?

Eventually, Sara found ways to move on. She made progress by:

1. ***Remembering a truth that's obvious but easy to overlook: we cannot change anyone but ourselves.*** We can try to influence, cajole, lecture, complain in front of them or behind their backs, but ultimately, no one will improve or change anything about themselves unless they want to. As we mature, we can try better tactics, such as being assertive and asking for what we need from others clearly and without being aggressive. But even then, we cannot guarantee that they can or will meet our needs. In the end, we must attend to ourselves.

2. ***Noticing where we are placing our attention.*** Sara understood that instead of focusing on her own work and her own behavior, she was concentrating on others' actions and problems. She also realized that as compelling as it was to focus on them, it was also a luxury. Unless Sara was blessed with boundless energy

and endless goodwill with her peers, she was choosing to tarnish her reputation and devote her most productive hours to addressing the shortcomings of the CEOs rather than doing her own work.

3. ***Knowing and doing our own work.*** Certainly, Sara knew her job description and what she was responsible for. But was she clear about her priorities? What were her most significant goals, and, equally important, how did she want to comport herself as she sought to achieve them? As she thought about her priorities, Sara did a mental evaluation of her progress. She considered whether she was advancing her projects as well as she had planned. She was also honest with herself about whether she was conducting herself like the leader she wanted to be.

Like many of us, Sara saw that there was room for improvement between what she *wanted* to achieve as a leader and what she *was* achieving as a leader. She saw that she was spending a lot of time thinking and talking about others' problems at the expense of her own effectiveness. That gap served as a wake-up call for Sara. She realized that she could refocus her attention and concentrate on closing that gap.

4. ***Last, think clearly about others' behavior and its effect on you.*** Sara thought carefully about the effect the CEOs' behavior had on her. Was she really hindered by the way they treated her? Was she truly a victim of their poor habits and lack of professionalism? Although she was mighty exasperated, Sara concluded that, in fact, their conduct did not interfere with doing her job. So, eventually Sara chose to reframe her view of their behavior as annoying irritations that she could live with and manage. She did not condone their actions, but she did affirm that she would always speak up for herself and ask for what she wanted. She also declared that she would no longer let her frustration about the CEOs distract her from doing her job and accomplishing her goals.

In the end, Sara realized that she had inadvertently abdicated her power as a leader and as a competent professional by concentrating on poorly behaving colleagues instead of concentrating on herself. She understood that her misplaced attention profoundly affected her productivity, work ethic, reputation, and career potential. Finally, Sara rededicated herself to focusing on her own work and nurturing her potential to become the outstanding nurse leader she knows she can be.

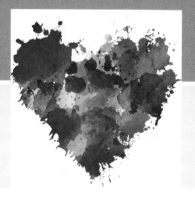

49

The Imposter Syndrome

"Sometimes I feel like a fraud." "If I am really honest, I am not sure if I belong in my leadership position. Do others wonder if I belong here too?" These instances of internal self-doubt are examples of the imposter syndrome. If you feel this way at times, you will benefit from understanding the imposter syndrome's effects, whether the seeds of doubt originate inside you or in your environment. Either way, how can you dim the shadow cast by the imposter syndrome so you can be the masterful leader you would like to be?

Our conference call was about to end. Just as this lively conversation among nurse leaders concluded, a participant said, "Can we talk about the imposter syndrome?"

The imposter syndrome? Of course we can talk about that! Since we were short of time, I decided to follow up privately with several participants, including Eve and Barbara. I want to offer you their perspectives, as well as those I gathered from my additional informal research on this topic. As you consider their definitions and views, I invite you to consider yours too. What do you think about the imposter syndrome? Have you experienced any version of it in your career? If so, what happened? How did you manage it?

Barbara is a very accomplished woman of color. She is articulate, commanding, well educated, and perceptive. Her comment about the imposter syndrome was direct and to the point: repeatedly, Barbara has felt that she has had to defend herself and her point of view. She believes she has needed extra credentials, more evidence for her decisions, and a willingness to work harder to achieve the recognition that comes more easily to others. Frequently, Barbara feels the leaders around her imply the question: "What are you doing in this role?" Still others convey a similar message: "Convince me that you deserve to hold this big job".

Barbara is not alone. As I spoke with other women leaders, they too expressed a similar "prove it to me" experience at some point in their careers. No matter what their ethnicity, women leaders often experience what sounds like a kind of hazing from other leaders when they enter positions of high authority. Many of these women spoke in the past tense, suggesting that as they grew in their roles and/or matured, this external "show me" attitude grew less common.

Now, let's turn to Eve. For many years, she says, she experienced the imposter syndrome too, but in a very different way. Eve is also an accomplished senior nurse leader. She is white, articulate, commanding, and well educated. For many years, she has been acknowledged as a leading authority in a particular area of health care leadership. However, for most of her career, Eve says she "felt like a fraud." She worried that she would be "found out," meaning that people might discover that she didn't really have all the answers—or at times, even some of the answers.

As I spoke with others about the imposter syndrome, I learned that they too had experienced this kind of internal self-doubt. Some felt that they had landed significant leadership roles because of their personalities rather than their abilities. Others realized that they appropriately doubted themselves; at times, it was right for them to question their competence. Who among us has not questioned our own capability when we are brand new to a role with significant responsibility?

What does the literature say? Much of the relevant research builds on the seminal work of Pauline Rose Clance and Suzanne Imes. As therapists at Georgia State University in 1978, they used the phrase "imposter syndrome" to describe the internal experience of a group of 150 high-achieving women in various fields who had a "secret sense" they were not as capable as others thought.[a] Through additional research, Clance and Imes also

---

[a]Clance P, Imes S. The imposter phenomenon in high achieving women: *dynamics and therapeutic intervention. Psychother Theor Res Prac.* 1978:15:241–247.

discovered that the syndrome didn't just apply to women. If men experience it, they may take steps to avoid having to show what they don't know.

What are the consequences of the imposter syndrome, whether it starts on the outside or the inside, or both?

- It can cause us to be moody and to experience performance anxiety that is disproportionate to our capabilities and/or the inherent challenges of our leadership roles.
- It can prompt us to "compete harder," which can lead to overpreparing and overworking. Habitually overworking leads to burnout, and overpreparing can suppress our capacity to be truly present and listen.
- It can force us to feel that good leadership is having the right answers rather than sometimes having the answers and at other times having the skills and courage to ask the right questions.
- It can distort the value of evidence, persuasion, "being right," and appearing invulnerable. While each of these has its place in effective leadership, taken together they can be overdone, much to the detriment of a leader who wants to be truly effective. It can stifle our interest in speaking authoritatively even when we are qualified. It can also discourage us from pursuing positions of greater responsibility and contribution.
- It can actually reduce the pressure on us by subtly influencing others to have lower expectations of us.

ALLEVIATING THE IMPOSTER SYNDROME

So, what can we do to mitigate the imposter syndrome?

- *Enlist the support of others, and find a mentor you respect and who respects you.* On a regular basis, share your experience of the imposter syndrome and solicit feedback.
- *Be aware of your self-talk.* Notice self-limiting thoughts and behaviors and unproductive conversation in your own head. Consider whether what you are saying to yourself is empowering or disabling.
- *Make a generous and realistic list of your own strengths.* Notice what you have to contribute. If this list described someone else, what would you think? How would you show respect for that person? How can you show that same level of respect for yourself?
- *Consider getting your list of strengths validated by others.*
- *Accept that "knowing it all" and other forms of perfection can be very costly pursuits.* Accept that no matter how hard we try, we will not be able to do everything perfectly.
- *Recognize that there are times when it is appropriate to assess that we are not as competent as we need to be.* In those cases, we need to seek new learning so our skills and knowledge better match our roles and responsibilities.
- *Be willing to be uncomfortable.* At times, we need to move through our fear and "do it anyway."

In the long run, many of us have grown out of the imposter syndrome and into our own knowledge and skills—and humility. We embrace what we know and all that we do not know. We are comfortable with the answers we have and the occasions in which asking others for input or help is the best strategy. Eve describes how she feels now that most days of the imposter syndrome are behind her: "I can now pull from all my experience and learning. I now feel more centered and balanced between what I know and what I don't know. But it has taken me many years to get to this place." Eve has gotten here by devoting time to self-care, reflection, and staying current with her learning edges and learning achievements.

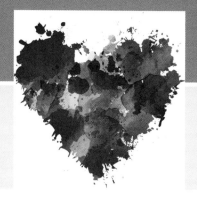

50

Keeping Expectations in Check

You are disappointed in how your colleagues are treating you. You want them to show more recognition for your good work, and your unmet expectations are affecting you emotionally. How can you confirm or let go of your assumptions and unverified beliefs about the meaning of your coworkers' behavior? How can you release the expectations that are not serving you and, in fact, are hurting you?

We know that there is a time and place for well-crafted expectations. For example, clear expectations are necessary components for leading a successful team. When the manager shares expectations with team members and those team members can ask questions, clarify, and sometimes renegotiate, both the manager and the team members are better able to fulfill their responsibilities.

But are we mindful of the role that expectations play in our many other professional interactions? This poignant question came to life when I heard two unrelated but strikingly similar stories. Camila and Ashley live in different parts of the country, and they are both smart, accomplished nurse managers who "know their stuff." By any measure, both Camila and Ashley are considered more than competent by their colleagues.

But both Camila and Ashley are challenged by their relationships with their bosses. In her years as a manager, Ashley has received consistently positive evaluations and support from all corners of her organization. But to her dismay, she has learned that her position is being eliminated. Although there is no certain date, she has known for months that she will be losing her job sometime in the next year.

Ashley has an intellectual understanding of the circumstances that led to the decision to end her employment. But she is having great difficulty emotionally accepting that her job will end. She is also having a hard time accepting how she was told about this very significant event.

The other manager, Camila, is not losing her job. But Camila feels that she has received little to no recognition for her contributions to her team's accomplishments. She says her boss does not acknowledge her for the articles she has written, awards she has won, and the consistent leadership she has shown both inside and outside the organization.

What do these situations, and the leaders who are in them, have in common? Here are a few similarities:

- Both Ashley and Camila are disappointed in how their respective supervisors are treating them, and they both want more recognition.
- Both are clear that if they were in their managers' shoes, they would do things differently. They would acknowledge and respect the successes that their subordinates have achieved, and Ashley says she would handle a valued employee's termination much differently.
- The realities of not feeling recognized for significant achievement and suffering a job loss are painful under any circumstances. But both Camila and Ashley are assuming that these actions are about being disrespected when disrespect may not be a factor in either of these situations. Just one possibility is that these supervisors do not know how to manage more effectively.

Both are aware of being angry and hurt, but neither can see that she is assigning meaning to her boss's actions that may not be accurate. They do not realize that their feelings are worsened by their unacknowledged expectations that their bosses will treat them the way they would treat others.

The story of outsized expectations is not just a story about Camila and Ashley. It is a story about many of us who have expectations that may not be conscious or spoken, but they are powerful enough to inflict real emotional distress on us and others.

There are many examples of ill-advised expectations. When we are harboring them, our internal dialogue might sound like one of these statements:

- My manager should manage the way I manage.
- If people behaved the way I would behave, they would treat me differently. They would ask my opinion and honor it—or they would at least listen and understand it when I offer it.

- When people hear what I have to say, or when they realize that they are approaching a situation incorrectly, they will see the light and admit that they are wrong.
- When people understand that "I am right," they will acknowledge me and the validity of my position.

MANAGING ILL-ADVISED HOPES

So what is the solution? Is there a remedy for misplaced expectations? It's very easy to say "just let them go," and if we can do that, life will surely be different. But for many of us, that is not so easy. Here are some ways to lessen our distress and become more effective.

1. *We can expand our self-awareness.* When others don't do what we want and we feel hurt, we can identify the true cause(s) of our hurt. Is it the actual situation (like Ashley's job loss)? Or is the way we are interpreting others' actions causing us to feel troubled for reasons that may not be accurate.
2. *We can be gentle and compassionate with ourselves.* The hurt that both Camila and Ashley feel is natural. But, as they become aware that their pain is amplified by their unspoken expectations of their bosses, they can see these expectations for what they are. In the process, they can honor and soothe their feelings of true grief and loss.
3. *We can own our part of the problem.* When we expect others to be excellent managers, and they are not, how can we deal with that in a way that is helpful?

4. *When our bosses do not behave as we would, even if we are "right," it is our responsibility to address that in a way that works.* To start, we need to objectively consider the facts rather than unintentionally filter those facts only through the lenses of resentment, hurt, and how "we would do it."
5. *We can consider what action, if any, we want to take.* Do we need to talk about what is occurring? Do we want to ask for something? As we become clear about problems that are ours to own, we can also become clear about what we will do to resolve or at least live with them more peacefully.
6. *If we are still having trouble letting go of ill-serving expectations, we can ask ourselves what it will take to release them.* To experience the benefit of this question, we need to be truly honest when we answer it.

I revisited Camila and Ashley recently, and both were more aware of what they had contributed to their problems with their bosses. They had both learned to focus less on the errors of their bosses' ways and focus more on proactively addressing their own challenges. Most important, both had learned that their natural emotional reactions had been unnecessarily intensified by their unstated and unfulfilled expectations of others.

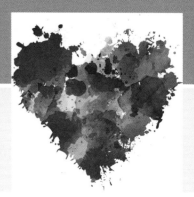

51

Take Advantage of Your Career "Runway"

Some strong leaders like to express themselves with great certainty. While exhibiting clear resolve can be a leadership asset, being too certain too often is not. Exhibiting too much certainty closes off new thinking and additional options. Thriving nurse leaders are discerning about when to be certain and when to be open to different perspectives that will generate choices rather than restrict them.

Maya is a skilled nurse leader with a substantial role in a hospital that is part of a large multistate health system. She is also a young mother with two children aged under 10 years. Maya's husband has a high-powered job that occasionally requires him to travel. Her position also involves some overnight travel, although Maya tries to keep it to a minimum.

Maya's supervisor Dennis sees a great deal of potential in Maya. In addition to supporting her participation in coaching and mentoring programs, he sponsors her efforts to obtain additional credentials and training in written and oral presentation.

Dennis regularly encourages Maya to move into a position with more responsibility. He is not prone to using superlatives, but Dennis has said that he considers Maya's potential leadership trajectory to be "unlimited."

For her part, Maya is ambitious and competitive, and she says that leadership challenges and opportunities energize her. However, she also says that "realistically, this is not the season (of my life) to pursue a senior leadership position." She is referring to her commitment to be fully present and engaged with her family as her children grow up.

Maya values Dennis' support and she also appreciates his lenience and understanding of her commitment to her family life. This has allowed Maya to excel in the role she has while maintaining enough flexibility to tend to her family's needs.

But recently, Maya's professional situation changed when Dennis announced his plan to retire in the coming year. This created an opening that would either be filled by someone else or Maya if she wanted to pursue moving ahead sooner rather than later. Dennis' colleagues on the senior team think highly of Maya, and she could be a strong contender for Dennis' job.

So, Maya had a decision to make—did she want to put her hat in the ring for Dennis' job or not? In fact, it didn't take Maya long to weigh the pros and cons of this choice; she quickly concluded that her children are still too young, so it is still "too soon."

Although that's a significant statement, this column is inspired by something else—that is, what Maya said next. Alluding to Dennis' system level leadership role, Maya said that she didn't want all the responsibility of Dennis' job. Then, she further said that, "I don't want my job to define me. I admire Dennis, but he has no life and he travels all the time. Although I am somewhat driven, I can't imagine doing that ever. So, I know I will never want a job like Dennis'."

This firm statement about Maya's future sounded alarm bells for me. Of course, I understood that her feelings were prompted by seeing Dennis have little to no personal time, and I could empathize with her air-tight conclusion that she didn't want that kind of existence.

But there was a problem. Although being clear is usually an asset, being so decisive now may not be wise for Maya. Why? Because she is needlessly restricting her professional options for many years to come. Such certainty about her ambitions far into the future will blind Maya to fresh, invigorating chances to upgrade her leadership experience and skills. These don't have to be "traditional progressively responsible positions." They could be less formal ventures that don't have to take a lot of time or be done alone. Such opportunities are often spotted by those who show initiative and demonstrate their willingness to address organizational issues—whether they are part of their formal job descriptions or not.

There is another consideration too. Tempting as it is, Maya does not need to exclude higher-level positions solely based on how others act in those roles. In fact, doing that would be unnecessary and career limiting. Although Dennis' lifestyle is not attractive to Maya, it is to some extent the way Dennis has chosen to perform his job. Dennis' approach to his role is not the only way to manage it, and we make a serious mistake if we assume that it is. Although there are givens in any job, there are also areas in which negotiation and customization are both possible and advisable.

Dennis has rightly observed that Maya has a "long runway." He is referring to her relatively young age and the many chances to experiment and learn that are in front of her. So, as Maya reflected on the circumstances of Dennis' departure, she took his comment to heart. She decided to leverage that "long runway" to her advantage, and she pulled back on her declaration that she would "never" be interested in holding a job like Dennis'. Instead, she considered different ways to practice and enrich her leadership skills while keeping an open mind about her future career choices.

Maya vowed to:

- *Seize the initiative when there is an unaddressed need that requires ingenuity and resourcefulness.* Such a need might constitute a special initiative or simply a one-time endeavor. Maya wants to "experiment" with activities like this so she can make a difference while learning whether she enjoys that kind of work.

- *Do her homework: when she sees these openings, she will learn the important facts, talk with the relevant stakeholders, and obtain permission before taking action.* Maya wants to be sure that there is a case to be made and support for expending the time and resources these efforts might require.

- *Volunteer to lead in different situations, so she can learn more about what she is good at and what she likes to do.* This will also give her the chance to see her shortcomings and become more skillful.

Maya's journey offers a valuable lesson to those with a "long runway" ahead. Even if it looks like the next job open to you is one you don't want or feel you are ready for, you can still grow and experience new ways of leading and learning by saying no to *only* this particular position. You can keep your long-term options open by being alert for other opportunities. When you say "yes" to those opportunities when they arise, you will nurture and prepare yourself for a meaningful leadership future—that is, the one you define and create for yourself.

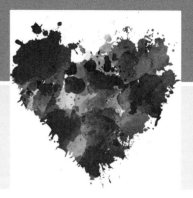

52

The Problem with Perfection

Some nurse leaders strive to perform perfectly on a day-in, day-out basis, and they find great fault with themselves when they don't. If they receive any negative feedback in the midst of otherwise glowing support, they will focus on this small part of the otherwise positive comments. What can we do to stop focusing on what's wrong? How can we right-size the impact of "negative" reflections, honor our disappointment, correct the problem, and move on? How can we be open to change and still celebrate what's right about our performance?

Jeff walked out of his supervisor's office feeling good mostly. He had just received his evaluation after a year on the job. Jeff is a nurse leader who holds a significant position in his health system, and he is very motivated to do well at work. He felt good because his review was very positive; on nearly every question with quantifiable measures, his manager said that he exceeded expectations. She awarded him the maximum salary increase even though the organization was facing difficult financial challenges. His manager's less-formal comments were largely positive too. She and the rest of nursing leadership realized the difficulty of Jeff's job, and he received high marks for his many achievements after just 1 year.

However, Jeff was disturbed by the comments his manager offered in the spirit of continuous improvement. She suggested that he delegate more and manage his own intensity so he wouldn't overpower others. She also said that, in her lengthy experience in the organization, it takes far more than 1 year to be truly effective in a role like Jeff's.

By the time Jeff and I spoke, a week had passed since his review. He started by telling me how positive the review had been, but he quickly steered our conversation to the parts he called "negative." As he spoke, I could hear increasing concern in his voice. I asked how his week had been since his review. He said that at the beginning, his wife wanted to celebrate with him and they'd had a great dinner out. Since then, he'd been unable to sleep and had been worrying about what his manager said about delegating and managing his intensity. He also mentioned that he had taken a couple of sick days to "avoid going to work."

Let's step back from Jeff's experience so we can learn from it. First, although his identity has been changed to protect his anonymity, this is a real situation and these are real responses. I offer Jeff's experience because it provides a good example of how hard we can be on ourselves when we do not receive a perfect score in our own eyes. By any measure, Jeff's review was exceptional. He also received honest feedback on how to improve his already impressive accomplishments.

Although Jeff heard the many positive comments, he focused on the few statements that he considered negative. They triggered him emotionally, and as his emotions took over, he lost perspective about the proportion and value of what was actually said. He began to believe that neither his manager nor he thought he was doing as well as he should at work. This story and his worry kept him awake at night. As he became more tired, he was less and less able to evaluate the quality of the feedback to determine whether it contained even a grain of truth. He began to feel badly physically too.

What was Jeff up to? Was he mentally or emotionally unstable? For our purposes, we're going to assume that Jeff is a capable and relatively emotionally healthy individual who, like all of us, has blind spots that can be managed. His particular blind spot is one that many of us share: *we are perfectionists, yet we are not perfect.* Events happen that we may interpret negatively, and then we believe our own "stories" and react to them.

In this case, Jeff's supervisor provided a performance review that was quite positive, a pay increase that could not have been larger, and a few comments to help Jeff grow. Jeff interpreted the latter comments as indicators of personal failure. He reacted by largely ignoring the positive feedback, not sleeping, and succumbing to the urge to hide by calling in sick.

It is very likely that, as a perfectionist, Jeff is unable to accept anything but perfect performance from himself and perhaps others. He has developed a bad habit over the years—emotionally reacting to his own interpretation of events without weighing the facts and without checking outside himself to see if his strong emotional reactions are warranted.

What are the costs of Jeff's perfectionism and his bad habit of interpreting and reacting, regardless of the facts? This behavior has an impact on:

- His efficacy at work, especially if he is prone to calling in sick
- His self-confidence on and off the job
- His ability to focus on what's actually happening and what's truly important versus what captures his attention emotionally

REVERSING A DOWNWARD EMOTIONAL SPIRAL

What is the remedy for Jeff and all of us who can be emotionally hijacked by events like these?

1. *Notice when we are emotionally triggered.* It takes practice, but the more we slow down to notice that we have been emotionally ensnared, the faster we are able to identify what the trigger was, evaluate how it's making us feel, and determine whether our reaction is warranted. We aren't striving to be emotionless; we are seeking to understand when our emotions take over and when we are not able to keep events and our reactions in proper proportion.

2. *Notice that when we start interpreting and telling ourselves a story (e.g., "my boss doesn't think I'm doing a good job"), our emotions grow stronger.* We become more upset. Notice that we are getting upset because of our own story, not because of what really happened.

3. *Notice that there are consequences when we start interpreting and telling ourselves (and perhaps others) stories about what happened instead of what actually happened.* For example, if Jeff had told his wife that his manager was disappointed in his performance, he

would have been telling her his story rather than what she actually said. His wife would have commiserated rather than celebrated. She might have even supported him in his need for time away from the job, and, just possibly, in a decision that he was going to leave the job. People who support us will be upset when we are upset; they will not want to hear that people don't value us. When we share these kinds of interpretations, we can garner lots of support that will salve our wounds. But this can actually do us a disservice. After we elicit outside support for our misinterpretations, we are less likely to step back and evaluate the accuracy of our initial reactions.

4. *Stop for a moment when we receive feedback that feels difficult.* Ask these questions: How much of this feedback is accurate? If this feedback is negative, does it contain any truth? Can we see how someone might say or feel this way?

5. *We need to ask ourselves whether we can let our emotional reaction go, once we have considered these questions and also experienced whatever our emotional reaction is.* Maybe we're not yet ready. That's fine as long as we recognize that we're reacting emotionally and should not take action (like stay away from work or even quit) as a result. Eventually, we'll be ready to more accurately gauge our next best steps.

6. *Realize that if we are perfectionists from way back, it may be difficult to stop reacting abruptly, no matter how disciplined we are.* We need to give ourselves permission to slip occasionally. Slips happen; when they do, it's important to restart our new practice of keeping feedback in perspective and ourselves on track.

As Jeff began to experience new ways of managing his reactions, he started feeling much better about himself, both on and off the job. Ironically, he learned to ask for and receive feedback about his performance on a frequent basis. He began to treasure constructive suggestions from those whose opinions he valued. His own self-esteem increased greatly. He became skilled at hearing and evaluating others' thoughts, feeling his own emotions, and not being enslaved by either.

Leading with Mastery and Heart

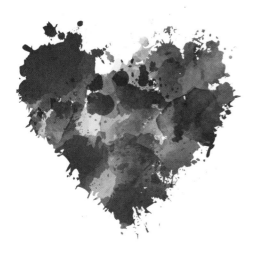

Nurses who lead with mastery and heart are exceptionally powerful. One source of their power is that they observe other leaders closely. They watch and learn from those around them, often seeing qualities they admire and choose to emulate. They also see ineffective behaviors and attitudes, and they consciously avoid these unsuccessful ways of leading.

Thriving nurse leaders know that others are watching them too. They are aware that they are models for the leaders and managers who see them from afar or close at hand. They understand the impact of their presence; they are aware that others observe them all the time, not just when they are "on stage."

What do others see in you that you want them to emulate? What would you like your leadership legacy to be? This final section highlights the ways in which you can leverage your mastery and heart to promote lasting growth in your colleagues and staff, and in your organization as well.

53

Grooming for All, Regardless of Budget

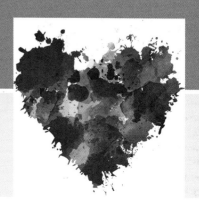

Nurse leaders need to develop and support those who are next in line for leadership. You know this, but can you do it when you have many other priorities and limited time? What if you don't have enough money to cultivate others' talent? This column shows that there are always ways to groom staff, even when budgets are limited or nonexistent.

Many nurse leaders say that they are committed to developing the next generation of leaders, yet many also say that they don't have the time or funds to help them grow. When you are working with talented staff with leadership potential, do you actively support them with concrete plans, engaging learning opportunities, and consistent follow-up?

If your answer to the last question is no, unfortunately, you are not alone. While there are robust leadership programs in some health care organizations, others are operating with organization-wide budget constraints and few available financial resources. So how do we groom talented leaders so that they are prepared to take the reins? How do we keep leadership development an actionable priority even in financially difficult times?

GROOMING DONE RIGHT

Not long ago, Lisa, an outstanding nurse leader, contacted our team regarding one of her organization's finest middle managers. Lisa described Belinda as a true star who was a bit rough around the edges. She was interested in executive coaching that would groom Belinda for senior leadership in this complex and highly regarded organization.

Although Lisa was appropriately cost conscious, she wanted Belinda to have a full complement of aids to promote her leadership growth. In concert with Lisa

and Belinda's immediate boss, the coach worked out a program that included regular coaching sessions; periodic sessions with Belinda and her peers, superiors, and/or direct reports; and occasional "shadow" coaching to observe Belinda in action. They also agreed on supplemental reading and assessments that would provide Belinda with 360° feedback and a measure of her emotional intelligence.

From the beginning of the engagement, Belinda's talents and potential were on full display and so was her attitude. She eagerly devoured the coaching sessions, the reading, and the between-session assignments. After each session, she shared her learning with her immediate boss. She thoughtfully absorbed the results of both assessments, including the portions that were not comfortable to hear. Belinda and the coach regularly discussed her progress with her immediate supervisor and Lisa.

Throughout her coaching, Belinda chronicled her insights and questions. She ended her coaching with a good understanding of her accomplishments, her remaining learning edges, and the path to sustain and expand her capacity as a leader.

GROOMING FOR THE REST OF US

You may be thinking that this is a nice story, but it's unrealistic for you and your organization. You can't make this kind of investment right now. If this is the case for you, what is there to learn from Lisa's ideal approach? What reasonable steps can you can take, even with real limits on your time and money?

To recognize these steps, let's move away from the specifics of Belinda's program so we can see less expensive options.

1. ***We need to be the mentors and role models we would want to have.*** Throughout her coaching, Belinda talked about how much she admired Lisa. For Belinda, Lisa embodied the best qualities of leadership. Belinda was learning every day just by watching her. We need to remember that the next generation of leaders is always watching us. Never underestimate the fact that you, and all of us, are on display all the time. We need to be the leaders that the next generation wants to emulate.
2. ***Recognize talent.*** Belinda benefited significantly from Lisa's mentorship. Although she was well above Belinda in the organization's hierarchy, Lisa recognized her talent and intentionally sought to develop her. Consider who you know who has potential and make it a priority to do whatever you can do to mentor and support them. Enlist the involvement of their immediate supervisors and others who can contribute to their growth.
3. ***Tell gifted individuals what you see in them.*** Lisa met regularly with Belinda before, during, and after her coaching program. She also provided clear and actionable feedback. Although most of Lisa's comments were positive, some targeted areas needed growth. These consistently candid reflections showed Belinda that Lisa saw her fully and added to the credibility of Lisa's comments.
4. ***Give talented individuals growth-producing resources inside or outside your organization, even if they are limited.*** In addition to providing her with an executive coach and a rigorous, customized learning program, Lisa encouraged Belinda to sign up for inexpensive in-house classes that would complement her coaching and deepen her repertoire of skills.
5. ***Promote the use of high-quality assessment tools.*** Well-chosen assessments can have a significant impact on a leader. Identify trained facilitators inside or outside your organization to maximize the value of these assessments. Appropriately debriefed assessments help leaders better understand their strengths and how they impact others. They also reveal blind spots the leaders might not see otherwise. One caution to be taken— when assessments are used in this context, the same assessments should not be used in performance reviews.
6. ***When you identify leaders with potential, consider how closely and frequently you can engage with them as they grow.*** In addition to Lisa's consistent involvement, Belinda's boss made it a regular practice to ask her what was happening in her coaching. This practice had many benefits, including helping Belinda stay accountable.
7. ***If you're not able to follow-up with gifted managers yourself, find others who can.*** Perhaps these are your own direct reports or they may be coaches or mentors inside or outside the organization. Wherever these resources are housed, their presence lets your mentees know that you care and that you are actively investing in their ability to excel.

During her coaching, Belinda frequently said that she felt supported by her organization and superiors. The fact that Belinda's immediate boss and Lisa were consistently willing to devote their time and money to her growth spoke volumes to her. She understood that the organization could not do this for every leader, and she did not want to squander any aspect of her good fortune.

Your protégés will also recognize your commitment to them. No matter how few fiscal resources you provide, they will still feel your support if you initiate and sustain nurturing actions that fit your circumstances. These may be the most important steps any of us can take to engage and inspire those who will follow in our footsteps.

54

The CNO as Chief Influence Officer

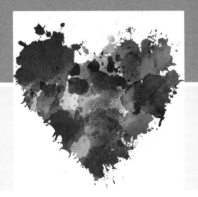

Your power to role model cannot be overstated. Here, the chief nursing officer (CNO) reveals to her staff her struggles with overwork, overeating, and excessive attention to taking care of others. Her example of vulnerability and candor helped to change her organization's nursing culture and improve the health of the managers who worked for her. She led the way for growth and learning for all, and in doing so she also received support for her own evolution as a masterful and thriving nurse leader.

I have the privilege of working with a team of 20 nurse leaders in a health care system that is undergoing change at all levels. In the past 18 months, they have experienced senior-level leadership transitions; new, high-profile community alliances; major service expansions; unpredictable census spikes; and the opening of a new hospital. They have also endured significant staff shifts and some reductions in force.

The leaders who remain have expanded scopes of responsibility and larger workloads. Some feel ill-prepared for the bigger roles they have been asked to assume. Undoubtedly, these leaders are stressed and exhausted. Yet, consistently, their behavior demonstrates a fierce commitment to their organization and especially to the patients they serve.

Although the team's determination to excel in this environment is noteworthy, their culture of self-care is the focus of this article. When I first encountered this group a few months ago, they looked world-weary. Their fatigue was palpable, and it was seeping into their interactions with each other, and probably with their patients and families too. *If they hadn't said they were worn out, I would have known anyway because the signs were so obvious.*

Here's what was happening:

- *Many, if not most, were working long hours for long periods of time.*
- *Many, if not most, were not exercising regularly or sleeping well.*

- *Some had daunting responsibilities at home and at work.* Their family challenges included illness, poor financial health, and difficult relationships. Others had professional challenges including charge nurses who were not prepared for their new roles and/or staff who were also exhausted from the effects of so much change.
- *Many were concerned that their staff would leave.*
- *Many, if not most, were discouraged by the amount and seemingly unending pace of major change.* They were trying to do the right thing, but they were disheartened because they could not catch their breath.

Deeper patterns were evident too, including the group's frequently articulated intentions to "do better" with self-care. But when circumstances at work didn't change, many abandoned those intentions. Then they felt worse.

Despite their CNO's interest in empowering the team to solve their own problems and to care for themselves, their capacity to manage their challenges was severely limited. They needed creative solutions, but their depleted states rendered them incapable of anything more than the basics. Their daily leadership choices were reactive rather than strategic and thoughtful.

This tableau may seem extreme, but the heavy weight of this team's responsibilities is not unusual. But what is noteworthy is what Danielle, the CNO, did about it.

First, she made a commitment to a multipronged, multi-month customized leadership development initiative for these leaders. However, it's not her commitment to "leadership development" that is chapter-worthy. What is worthy of our attention is the influence Danielle wielded when she stepped forward and spoke candidly about her own self-care demons.

In the team's first retreat, Danielle took the floor. In less than 10 minutes, she talked about her lifelong habits of working too hard and making herself constantly available. She reflected on eating too much and exercising too little. She also shared what she was learning about herself. She told the team that when left unchecked, these behaviors were destructive to her and those around her. She owned the fact that her ways of leading had contributed to a culture of overwork, excess stress, and, ultimately, a less than fully productive workforce.

Danielle went on to candidly share what she was doing to reverse course, including working fewer hours, getting more exercise, improving her nutrition, and setting a better example for all who looked to her for leadership, including those in the room.

Danielle concluded her brief talk by telling the team to get their work done and then take time away from their jobs. She explicitly gave them permission to "leave the building and go home." She specifically said, "It's not about being here all the time."

These words may sound simple, but she meant them, and they were potent. When I returned to the system 5 weeks later, I learned that as many as half of the team left right after that offsite meeting. They covered their bases, but they didn't return to the hospital until the next day—and the retreat ended at 1:00!

What followed was even more significant. Danielle didn't just say these words once. In the months that followed, she modeled them. She demonstrated that her commitment to her own self-care was real. She had always worked long, long hours, but she cut them back. She also stopped sending non-urgent e-mails on weekends and late at night.

Danielle has followed through on her personal commitment to better health, and as the months have gone by, the results of her newfound regimen are unmistakable. Her promise to support the team's self-care for the long haul is evident too. She regularly asks the team how they are doing with their own self-care strategies. And here are just two of the outcomes:

1. When a few of the team members made commitments to exercise more, work shorter hours, and eat properly, many others did the same thing. Danielle's permission-giving and behavioral examples reverberated throughout the team. The leaders weren't just following Danielle's lead, they were following each other.

2. What started as self-care in the literal sense grew into self-care in the broader sense. Most of the team members report that they are saying "no" more often. They are also speaking up frequently; getting organized and staying organized; and teaching partners and direct reports what they need to know and holding them accountable for doing it.

This did not begin as a formal study, so these results were not measured. But it is clear that these leaders and those around them are benefiting from the wonderful results this dedicated team has created. As they go forward, the team's members are supporting themselves by helping each other stay on track and providing support when they go astray.

As Danielle predicted, the rate and amount of change are not slowing for this health care organization. The environment in which these leaders operate is the same, but the team is not. Now, they create and implement strategies to live with and even excel when the demands are stressful.

Danielle's efforts to inspire and the team's commitments to better their self-care are not perfect. Their good intentions to leave earlier, eat well, and sleep enough are not always realized. But this team and their leader have been successful enough. When I work with them now, I am partnering with awake, engaged leaders who are eager to learn and practice new skills and behavior. Their "culture change" is real, not perfect, and their momentum is real too. And they show no signs of slowing down.

55

Turning Poor Performance Around

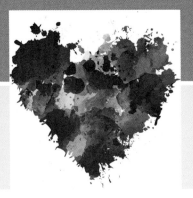

Your direct report isn't doing well and you are disappointed in him. You've talked with him about your concerns, but there has been no significant change in his behavior. You are aware that if this performance pattern continues, you will lose this employee either because he quits or you fire him. How might you unwittingly be contributing to his lack of success?

Laurie is challenged with finding and keeping good managers. As a vice president of a community health system, she understands the critical importance of this leadership function. Yet, despite her other strengths, Laurie is consistently unable to groom, guide, and evoke the best from the gifted nurses who report to her.

Laurie knows that this personal challenge poses a serious threat to her future success, and she wants to tackle the problem with a fresh approach. Specifically, she wants to know how to deal with her concerns about Marita's performance. Marita is a nurse leader who Laurie admired enough to hire and relocate after an extensive search. At the time, Laurie described Marita as the perfect fit for the position.

Now after 2 years, Laurie sees things differently. She is no longer sure Marita is going to make it, and her second performance review is coming up. It is Laurie's practice for direct reports to complete their own reviews before they meet, and she thinks that Marita will give herself high ratings.

Laurie's view about Marita's conduct is different. Although Marita excels at the community functions that are central to her work, Laurie says she demonstrates below-average skill with organization and planning. Furthermore, Laurie believes that Marita is not able to set priorities, meet deadlines, focus on details, and communicate well in writing.

Laurie knows that she needs to pause before she has the meeting with Marita. If she simply proceeds, it is likely that Laurie will lose another valued employee.

Laurie's situation is familiar for many of us. We feel strongly, we are about to act, but we know we may be making a big mistake. Although Laurie has a bias toward action, in this case she stopped herself. She did not simply react to her strong negative feelings. Instead, she sought outside help and managed a significant change within herself. Consequently, she moved from nearly firing Marita to getting her point across *and* becoming genuinely engaged with Marita's view of her work.

What happened? How did Laurie make such a dramatic shift? First and most important, she was willing to get outside of her own head by seeking counsel from someone who would respect and also challenge her thinking. Second, Laurie was willing to redirect her focus; she stopped thinking so much about Marita and started thinking more about herself. By exploring what was going on within herself, Laurie learned that:

- She had not considered how she was contributing or not contributing to Marita's lack of success.
- She was repeating a pattern she had played out with other direct reports many times.
- She was experiencing the same strong negative judgments she felt when other staff leaders did not have these strengths.

Luckily, Laurie could see the patterns that emerged. She wanted to know why she ended up in the same conversation with so many of her direct reports. She also wanted to learn how her performance management challenges related to emotional intelligence (EI). Most important, she wanted to know what to do with what she learned.

The most telling piece of information is that consistently Laurie discovers the same shortcomings in many of the managers who report to her. Without fail, she becomes upset when others do not or cannot excel with organization, detail, and planning. An equally compelling piece of information is that these perceived shortcomings in others are exceptional strengths for Laurie. She believes that her own outstanding abilities in these same areas provide her with a commanding sense of control.

However, by repeatedly finding fault with these skills in others, Laurie is exhibiting, over and over, an excessive need for control. As Laurie considered this insight, she said that she has been called overly controlling for years. She volunteered that this is probably driven by old messages and her fear of failure on the job.

UNDERSTAND THE NEED FOR EMOTIONAL SAFETY

The literature on EI tells us that such fear can be propelled by our hard-wired human need to stay emotionally safe. As Laurie considered how this reality applied to her, she grew close to the heart of her challenge: How could she manage her employee's performance in an emotionally intelligent way? What would that look like in the meeting with Marita?

From an EI vantage point, *Laurie's real work is to become aware of her own need for emotional safety and:*

- *Notice how it can drive and, at times, sabotage her intentions and behavior, especially if it remains unconscious*
- *Actively manage her quest for safety in ways that promote rather than inhibit productive relationships with others*

But, how does she do this? First Laurie considered the cost of letting her wishes for control and safety overwhelm her other thoughts and feelings. She realized that her unwitting needs had closed off access to her appreciation of Marita's strengths. For example, although she would allude to Marita's accomplishments in passing, Laurie usually followed such recognition with the word *but*. Laurie learned that this word effectively cancels out any previous acknowledgment of Marita's strong points.

Laurie's need for control and safety also closed off her curiosity about Marita's vision for herself in the position. Before pausing to examine her own internal state, it did not even occur to Laurie to ask about Marita's view of the future: What did Marita want to achieve for the community she served? What did she want to achieve for their organization? What did she want to achieve for herself?

When Laurie explored her feelings, she began to appreciate again why she hired Marita in the first place. Laurie's honest reflection paid a valuable dividend: she made a significant emotional shift that allowed her to have an entirely different dialogue with Marita. She led from a position of genuine curiosity and appreciation instead of negative judgment. After their meeting, Laurie reported that:

1. She started the conversation by recognizing Marita's accomplishments and asking about Marita's vision for her position and for herself.
2. She was curious about Marita's future goals; what did she really want to achieve in her professional life?
3. She focused on actively listening to Marita's aspirations.
4. Together, they spent most of the meeting aligning Marita's ambitions with the overall vision for the health system.
5. As the conversation flowed, Laurie made suggestions that supported Marita's growth. At the same time, Laurie made valid points about the skills she wanted Marita to strengthen (organization, follow through, etc.). She placed her expectations in the context of Marita's vision, the organization's goals, and what Marita needed to work on to be successful.
6. Laurie sensed that Marita fully listened and took in each of her requests.
7. Laurie kept tabs on her own feelings. She observed herself listening with an open mind and an open heart. As she did this, Laurie believed that Marita's engagement in the conversation grew stronger. In turn, Laurie's own enthusiasm grew too. As they talked together, Laurie reengaged her own vision for their work on behalf of their community and its health. She became reinvigorated with her original excitement about what they could achieve together.

In the end, both Laurie and Marita said they were very satisfied with the discussion. In fact, Laurie was so energized that she remains enthusiastic about Marita's work to this day.

56

Does Anyone Want Your Job?

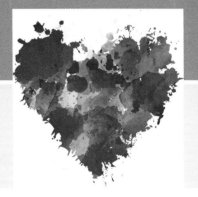

You are a leader and manager. You work hard, achieve great results, and make a good salary. But, does anyone want your job? If not, why not? Here, we focus on what others see that we may not see about how we are occupying our positions. We also focus on ways we can inspire rather than repel others who will eventually be candidates for our positions.

It never fails. When I teach aspiring nurse leaders about leadership and coaching, no matter what the setting, there are charge nurses and managers who say that they don't want their supervisors' positions.

What about you? Does anyone want your job?

Of course, leadership roles are not for everyone. Still, there are too many qualified nurses who are reluctant to pursue leadership roles. How do we address this issue? I know you share concerns about developing future nurse leaders, because of the many queries I receive. Here are just a few examples:

- How do we ensure competency as we bring people forward?
- How do we encourage aspiring nurse leaders to challenge physicians when it is in the best interest of patient care?
- How do we prepare staff for leadership positions? What are some strategies to help them with the transition? What if they do not want these roles?

Succession planning is clearly on your minds. You are managing perpetual nursing shortages and the broader demographic challenges of today's workforce. You are keenly aware of the important task of replacing yourselves. You know one of your central challenges is to equip tomorrow's leaders with the skills they need to succeed, prosper, and lead satisfying professional lives.

Here we focus on just one element of this challenge: how you can best fulfill your responsibility to develop future nursing leaders. *Formally*, you and other readers occupy all types of positions that support succession

planning. Yet, there is one element of succession that every reader has in common: you occupy the most important seat in the house when it comes to the *informal* aspects of developing leaders.

OWN THE POWER OF YOUR ROLE

By definition, you possess an enormous capacity to influence whether the talent and contribution of your nursing colleagues come to fruition through leadership. By definition, you are a *role model*. You may not want that job, but it is yours anyway! Because you are a leader, you are watched at every turn. By definition, you positively or negatively influence those around you through the example you set.

You are also in a position to guide, mentor, coach, and facilitate the growth of others, no matter what your formal role in the hierarchy. *You* are the most important part of your organization's succession strategy. *You* have the greatest impact on those who are thinking about whether leadership is in their future.

The nurses who report to you look to you not only for answers and supervision but also for the truth about leadership. They look to you for a daily example of what leadership is really like. They learn about leadership through what you say, what you do not say, and the tone you set. They learn about leadership by observing and interacting with who you are *being* as a leader.

There is a great deal of power in your role. You have the opportunity to shape the future of your organization and the fields of nursing and health care leadership through your actions.

Here are some questions to consider as you reflect on this responsibility and your chance to bring engaged, prepared leaders into the world:

- ***How are you caring for yourself as a leader?*** What do you do to inspire, renew, and replenish yourself? Do you seek the support you need to attend to your own professional and personal needs?

- *How can you encourage, support, and provide appropriate resources for those who will succeed you?*
- *How can you assist staff to accurately assess their leadership learning needs?* Do you tell your staff about the talent and potential you see in them? Do you give them guidance about how to increase their leadership effectiveness?
- *How can you provide sufficient safety so that potential leaders will speak honestly with you about their concerns?* Do you really listen when they raise questions about their future quality of life, compensation, or ability to participate in direct patient care?

- *How can you help your organization create a culture that future leaders will want to embrace?*

If you work with nurses who are new to leadership roles, do you give them what they most need in the early stages of their leadership journey? Do you provide them with opportunities to learn the skills and competencies they must have to succeed? Do you offer them support so they can experiment and practice their new behaviors?

Indeed, you are in the driver's seat when it comes to leadership succession. How can you prepare and nurture yourself so that you bring your best spirit and talent to the task?

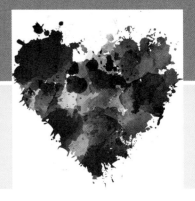

57

Coach While You Lead

The power of coaching as a leadership development strategy is well documented. Should you be a coach or hire a coach for your team? While taking these steps will maximize the impact of coaching in your organization, you as a masterful nurse leader can learn and practice basic coaching techniques that will enhance the work of those you lead. This is the first of two chapters about coaching tips (and traps) for thriving nurse leaders.

Recently, I had the honor of working with a team of nurse leaders who are eager to incorporate coaching skills into their everyday work. Their learning journey offers valuable lessons for us all.

We know that coaching has "come of age" in health care and nursing leadership in recent years. In countless health systems, coaching is no longer considered punitive or the sole province of poor performers. In fact, in many venues, coaching is a reward for good performance and increased leadership responsibility.

These statements refer to formal coaching, meaning engagements in which an internal or external professionally trained coach is made available to a manager or leader. What about "everyday" coaching for the rest of us? Should we care about incorporating "everyday" coaching skills into our portfolio of management capabilities? Yes! Here are just three of many reasons:

1. In our field, big changes are here and more are coming. We must all adapt to remain effective, but for some employees, adjusting is not easy. Leaders with a genuine interest in obtaining coaching skills can facilitate meaningful dialogue and learning in others. These efforts forge stronger bonds that help staff members stay engaged as they manage profound shifts in their work.
2. The "war for talent" is back. This term was first coined by McKinsey and Co. in their now-classic book.[a]

---

[a]Michaels E, Handfield-Jones H, Axelrod B. *The War for Talent*. Cambridge, MA: Harvard Business Review Press; 2001.

Although much has changed since then, today's war for talent is just as real. Why? Chief among the reasons is that skilled, ambitious workers have a broad array of work options. For health care organizations, employee engagement is not just a good idea; it's imperative if we want to grow and keep our people.

3. Even if the war for talent weren't back, the cost of employee disengagement and turnover is not going down. We continue to sacrifice millions in lost productivity when employees are not using their full complement of skills and energy.

PRACTICE FOUNDATIONAL COACHING SKILLS

So, what are some basic coaching skills that foster growth and engagement with others? In my experience, using just these few behaviors provides significant benefit for all:

- *Communicate clearly and openly.* The focus here is on asking open-ended questions and listening genuinely to the answers. Humans are best equipped to listen openly when we are not judging the person or their comments before they are uttered. Leaders can learn a lot when we stop asking yes or no questions and start asking sincerely curious questions that start with "how" or "what." This is not to suggest that all conversations with employees need to eliminate judgments and be curious questions that start with these words. Leaders are paid for their judgments, but those judgments are very limiting when they are the only tools in the toolbox.
- *Monitor yourself.* When we coach, we need to be mindful of who we are "being" in the conversation. I mentioned judgment above, but we also want to consider whether we are projecting our answers or our own situations onto our coaching partner (the "coachee"). Are we projecting how we would feel if we were the other person? Are we making assumptions about what their actions mean? These questions are always important, but as we become more sensitive to diversity and its

many dimensions, monitoring our own projections and assumptions moves to center stage when we coach.

- *Understand resistance.* It's helpful to remember that resistance is normal. Change of any size is not easy for many people, and as managers, it is beneficial to "normalize" pushback before we start to resist the resisters. From a coaching standpoint, our job as a manager is to understand the resistance and to help employees move through it so they can become more engaged and productive. Understanding resistance is most often achieved by being curious and listening. When we do these things, we may learn something important about the change, and we will certainly learn something important about the individual who is resisting. No matter what, we will want to attend to the resistance. Left to its own devices, resistance can become toxic to the individual and the team—resisters love to enroll others so they have company in their state of discontent.
- *Move ahead.* Coaching is not coaching if there is no active component. What is the follow-up? What is your coachee going to practice or do differently, even just once, as a result of your conversation? Help your coachee grow by encouraging him or her to try something new. Be an accountability partner (if you wish) and set up a follow-up conversation to see how the experiment went. Support success if it went well. Be patient if it didn't.

KNOW THE PITFALLS

Here are a few pitfalls to be aware of when you coach.
1. *Notice whose agenda you are coaching.* As manager, it may well be yours, and if it is, be transparent with your coachee about this. Sometimes novice coaches lead with their own agenda, but they ask questions that suggest they want to work with the coachee's agenda. This can be confusing for the coachee, at best, and at worst, it will be perceived as insincere and manipulative.
2. *Watch for "overtelling."* In my experience, most nurse leaders have a well-developed muscle named "I have the answer." This well-toned capacity is vital to the role of nurse leader. But, like any strength, this one can be overused when we are coaching to facilitate growth and learning in others.
3. *Be patient.* Some leaders say they are natural coaches. That may be true, but being curious, not leading with judgments, and not telling run counter to the work that many leaders do every day. When we are learning a new skill, it is easy to become frustrated with ourselves and revert to old behaviors. Don't worry; with coaching as with many other skills, practice makes us a lot better.
4. *Coaching is not a hammer and every problem is not a nail.* When managers learn to coach, they often try coaching out on every challenge. Although it is perfect for many situations, coaching is not the solution for everything a leader encounters.

If you are already on the road to using good coaching skills in your work, congratulations! If you are just starting out, good luck and best wishes. Coaching is a skill worth honing.

58

Let Coaching Fill Your Heart

This is the second of two chapters about how nurse leaders can develop others by serving as their leader coach. This piece offers more coaching tips, and it also discusses the great emotional and psychic rewards of coaching those who want to grow in their stewardship roles.

What do the terms "coaching" and "mentoring" mean in your organization? Do they suggest discipline or do they convey growth and support?

Regardless of how these terms are defined in your setting, it is likely that your leadership role calls for your active involvement in the growth of others. When we partner as mentors and coaches with our staff, we become "leader coaches." When we serve in this way, we can become welcome sources of knowledge, skill, inspiration, and encouragement. Our learning partners can develop trust in us as advisors and creators of a safe space so they can practice difficult conversations and new behaviors, share concerns, and explore fresh ways of managing and leading. Once we have earned their trust, we can provide mirroring and insight they might not receive otherwise.

These learning partnerships are critical for leadership success, and just one reason is that nurse and health care leaders at all levels crave feedback. Needing thoughtful and objective feedback isn't just the province of younger, less experienced leaders. It's a truism, but for most of us, the higher we go, the less feedback we receive. As a "trusted advisor," you can offer feedback and many other gifts to your learning partners.

What about your own growth? Is the business of being a leader coach a one-way street? Certainly not! For example, if your staff has become more skilled because of your guidance, that could be reward enough. You could even say that the purpose of your coaching has been achieved.

But many leaders know that mentoring and coaching others also give us "psychic and emotional" benefits. Just one is that we witness the beauty of the human spirit when

it is "tended." When we intentionally engage as mentors and coaches, we take the time to see the world from another's point of view. And when it's called for, we share a slice of what we understand about that person's world, and we offer perspective about how they operate within it.

Within the trusting container of the relationship we create together, our learning partners can stop and think. They can ask themselves honest questions like, "Is this how I want to show up?" or "What have I forgotten to pay attention to, own and/or share that changes the picture?" As leader coaches, we can ask how our partners see their circumstances differently than we do. Or, we can stimulate their imaginations with fresh views as they reflect and craft their visions for moving forward.

These conversations are rich dialogues in which we as leader coaches witness the commitment and vulnerabilities of our partners. We learn that we can maintain our own perspectives while also being enriched by others. We can also be challenged by unexpected ideas that force us to open our minds and leave the comfort of our own "box." The learning goes both ways.

We may know our managerial roles very well, but do we know how best to engage as leader coaches? What areas of expertise do we need to sharpen so others can blossom into the leaders they are capable of being? In turn, what capacities will help us be more successful on our own journey to leadership excellence?

SUBTLE BUT IMPACTFUL COACHING SKILLS

Here are a few skills that will go a long way toward these ends:

- *As leader coaches, our greatest gifts are our presence and attention.* Coaching and mentoring don't have to take a lot of time, but they do require some. After all, we are investing in others and in ourselves. It's a two-way investment. We can even consider it an act of self-care.

- *We want to be conscious and deliberate as we fulfill this role.* From the "leader coach" stance, our job is to listen, respect, and offer ways in which our partner can develop. It is our responsibility to understand, mirror, and gently challenge when that's appropriate.
- *We need to be honest with ourselves when we have negative judgments or feelings about the "coachee."* If we feel that way consistently, we are not the right coach for this individual. But if our disapproval is sporadic, it's worth asking ourselves if we can get beyond these occasional feelings. Can we be open, and do we want to better understand this person? Are we willing to let go of assumptions that may be incorrect? If we can do this, we can shift from being negative to wanting to learn more. We can ask curious, open-ended questions that will enable us to see our learning partner more clearly. We also may be able to better recognize our own biases.
- *As "leader coaches," we can fulfill these responsibilities when we enter the dialogue refreshed and aware that we are there to be of support.* We may truly want what's best for the other person, and in that case we are relatively "agenda-free." Or we may have an agenda such as wanting this individual to lead more effectively or take on more responsibility. In that case, we can own our goal, and at the same time acknowledge and honor that the other person is in charge of their own path.
- *Finally, we can let go of our commitment to "being right."* As I have described elsewhere,[a] attachments to having the right answer come naturally when we are skilled, experienced, and bright. But being convinced we are right does not serve us or anyone else when it prevents us from hearing other points of view and listening with respect. As effective coaches and mentors, we succeed when we offer guidance *and* allow others to find their own voice, whether that voice is the same or different from our own.

Mastering these skills can take a lifetime of practice, but it's worth it. Your impact cannot be overstated: your colleagues can flourish with your help, and your hearts can truly fill with joy.

---

[a]Robinson-Walker C. *Leading Valiantly in Healthcare: Four Steps to Sustainable Success.* Indianapolis, IN: Sigma Theta Tau International; 2013.

59

What Are You Passing on to Others?

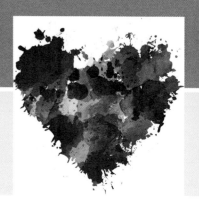

Exceptional nurse leaders have a lot to teach us. This piece focuses on a truly remarkable leader and how she influenced those who worked with and for her. It also highlights what she did to take care of her greatest leadership assets: her personal well-being and knowledge of what held heart and meaning for her.

A hospital in which I have spent a lot of time is undergoing major funding cuts. This community resource is part of a small health system, and it has earned a great reputation, especially in recent years. Today, its leaders are making every effort to maintain its quality of care while taking anything remotely "excessive" out of its budget.

I have worked with many of this organization's nursing leaders, and I can attest to their skill, persistence, and commitment to doing their very best work. They are an impressive group. Much as I would like to attribute their fine contributions to their innate leadership knowledge or even wisdom they have enhanced as a result of our work together, I believe that the largest portion of their success is due to another factor altogether.

Their chief nursing officer is a fantastic role model. Before I even met Courtney, I knew this about her. I could tell by the way people talked about her. My introduction to the hospital was through another senior leader who continually made reference to Courtney. I heard how universally she was revered in the organization, by the nurses and the other departments. I couldn't help but notice that she seemed to be on a pedestal. So when I was about to meet her for the first time, I was quite curious.

When I arrived in her office, I was greeted by a gracious and to-the-point executive. Courtney was welcoming and quite supportive of the leadership work to which we were all committing for the coming months. I was impressed enough in that first session, but it wasn't until later that I truly appreciated why she had earned the respect of nearly all the leaders around her.

It was true that Courtney espoused most of the adages we hear about leading others in turbulent times: foster great collaboration; encourage innovation; use the lessons of the present, past, and future; retain talent; and the like. But was this what was so special about Courtney? Was it really her way of working with others that was remarkable? I was skeptical. I wanted to learn much more about her leadership style.

MANAGING YOURSELF DURING STRESSFUL TIMES

I was fortunate enough to work closely with her and her team for several months, and I got to know what was unique about Courtney's approach to managing in difficult times. In addition to using proven best practices for managing people in tough times, *she paid equal attention to how she managed herself.*

Courtney knew that her very presence dramatically impacted those around her. Here are some of the ways in which she managed herself during times of significant stress for her managers, the staff, and the whole organization.

She let her values guide her. She knew what was important, and she imparted that message consistently to her team. As an example, when difficult budget decisions had to be made, Courtney relied heavily on her values and those of the organization. She encouraged her team members to do the same. After all, her team members were producing wonderful results for their patients;

Courtney had complete trust in the values of the leaders in her circle.

She managed her own fear. Courtney was experiencing personal financial challenges that were similar to those of her direct reports, and she did what she could to actively manage them. She realized that if she gave a lot of her attention to fear, it would escalate and consume her energy. She knew she needed to focus on managing the *hospital's* most significant challenges, so she did not give in to worrisome news that was outside of her control.

She managed others' fear, to the extent that anyone else can do that. She did this by telling the truth about what the organization was facing. In the months of my work with Courtney and her team, I never heard her mince words or put varnish on a difficult message. She simply told the truth. At the same time, she had a positive approach to that truth. Often her words were simple: "We can do this." Courtney resolutely believed in the organization's ability to perform, even in the most trying of times. When she said "We can do it," there was no doubt that she meant it.

She did her best to manage and remain conscious of her own internal "leadership seductions." These could also be thought of as manifestations of her "shadow," that dark side we all possess. She knew that the best antidotes were enough sleep, self-care, and forgiveness for others and herself. Courtney's intention was to take full ownership of the aspects of her life she could control while letting the rest go. For her, examples of these seductions were easy to spot: she might experience an impulse to be curt with others who weren't able to move ahead positively, or she might feel impatient with people who were impeding rather than enhancing progress. She might even be angry with other hospital leaders who were unable to stay focused on their vision of providing high-quality health care.

She paid attention to shifts in her own mood. Courtney was familiar with what Rick Maurer mentioned in his newsletter, "Leading in Turbulent Times."[a] In times of stress and pressure, it is important to pay attention to what Maurer calls "the weather," or shifts in organizational conditions that can change quickly. Courtney heeded this guidance as it applied to others in the organization and as it applied to her. She realized that manifestations of her shadow could emerge from time to time. Courtney resolved to notice this tendency and manage it when it surfaced.

She did her best to grow comfortable with "not knowing." She focused on becoming at ease with ambiguity, learning in the moment, and making prompt decisions with enough—if not perfect—information. She also gave explicit permission for the nurse leaders that reported to her to do the same.

Courtney would not want to see herself painted with a brush that suggests perfection. In a way, her greatest strength is her ability to be aware of, learn from, and grow with her own imperfections. Most of the people with whom she works don't know that she focuses on managing these parts of herself. What they do know is how she shows up every day in the organization and how she relates as their leader. At the beginning, I said that her team members admire her. That's because Courtney is the kind of leader that many of our organizations need now, more than ever. I firmly believe that, in our own individual ways, we all have the potential to lead just as effectively as Courtney does.

---

[a]Maurer R. Leading in turbulent times. 2008. http://www.beyondresistance.com/LeadingToday.pdf. Accessed March 16, 2009.

60

Develop Your Unique Leadership Style

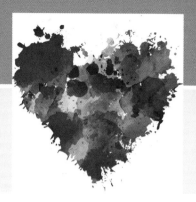

Leadership authenticity and presence are qualities that are difficult to define but palpable when we experience them. The thriving nurse leader featured in this chapter has an artful and unique leadership approach. Here, we take a look at the leadership behaviors and attitudes she employs to manage her many responsibilities and professional relationships.

There is something exceptional about Grace. She is a nurse executive with whom I have worked for several years, and recently she applied for and was promoted to the chief executive officer (CEO) role.

Although she was delighted, Grace was somewhat taken aback by her colleagues' choice. Her surprise was not an expression of immodest (and perhaps false) humility. Rather, it was a statement of curiosity—what led the leaders of this esteemed tertiary facility to select her?

Although Grace was a bit startled, I was not. As her leadership coach, I have seen examples of her potent ability on many occasions, and I'd like to share her approach with you. I am convinced that the essence of Grace's leadership strength is available to each of us. Regardless of our roles, all of us possess the capacity that she has truly mastered. It is her heart-full and unique leadership presence.

For Grace, this means that she is aware of herself as a grounded and powerful individual, and she is intentional about continuing to understand her strengths, challenges, and influence as a leader. She regularly exhibits her willingness to be a learner. This decision keeps Grace current with the impact of her talents. It also allows her to be at choice; she can skillfully select her approach to given situations in her work.

Grace has an artful leadership style that is based on honest self-assessment, feedback, practice, and acceptance of her own abilities. It is certainly true that Grace has the requisite skills, knowledge, and experience that technically qualify her to be a senior leader. But that is not what is most compelling about her. We all know individuals who are technically qualified yet not strong and successful leaders. What is compelling about Grace is that she effectively integrates ongoing learning as she relaxes into being who she is.

AN EXAMPLE OF ARTFUL STYLE

Let's get specific about some of the ways Grace demonstrates this quality. First, let me offer several caveats. In isolation, none of these behavioral images does Grace justice. Second, it is the combination of these approaches that makes her an exceptional leader. Third, these descriptive comments may make Grace seem superhuman. That is certainly not true. On some level, writing this or any example lifts Grace's presence out of reality and places it into the realm of "study."

That said, let's move ahead. In each interaction between Grace and other hospital leaders, I see her adept approach to creating and managing relationships. She collaborates effectively with the many others upon whom the organization depends for its success. When she engages with peers, subordinates, and other senior leaders, ***Grace is clear, to the point, warm, open, inviting, and decisive.***

She is also steady and respectful; I have never seen Grace appear arrogant or treat others with anything less than complete dignity. She has an uncanny ability to understand organizational dynamics and work with others in ways that leave them both enabled and inspired.

Here are other ways in which Grace exhibits her artful style:

- ***She is genuine with herself and others.*** The people with whom she interacts perceive her to be real, and this quality invites and builds their trust. They may not like every position she takes, but they take her at her word. Grace is right-sized and clear about who she is. In other words, Grace is genuine, and that is a natural part of her fabric as a human being. It is also a strategic choice. She knows that people respond well and on a deep level to integrity in a leader.

- *She does not overly distort what she says or hears.* Although some filters are inherent in all of us, Grace does a skillful job of managing hers. She has made it a point to develop awareness about the biases and experiences that shape her beliefs and values. She does her best to remain aware of these influences. In other words, she vigorously manages herself.
- *Grace listens to understand and intentionally reflects on what she has heard.* She actively monitors the stories she tells herself. She is diligent in her efforts to accurately represent her own or others' actions and intentions. She takes care to avoid misrepresenting others and herself. Grace is also committed to withholding judgment until she has enough information to make informed decisions.
- *Grace is not overly focused on herself;* therefore, she is available to pay more attention to those around her.
- *Grace believes in self-renewal.* This was not always so. She was always a hard worker, and assuming the role of CEO demanded nothing less. After an initial period of intense 12-hour and longer days as the new CEO, she found that she was less energetic than normal. She decided to pare her work week from 60-plus hours. As she implemented this difficult choice, she was not unrealistic. Sometimes working less is not possible. But whenever it is, she does it. Every few weeks, she takes a day away from the office to work at home. She schedules vacation time, gets sufficient sleep on most nights, engages in regular exercise, and is learning to meditate. Most of us recognize the difficulty of combining organizational leadership with personal well-being. These are not easy commitments to keep, but Grace is disciplined about making exceptions. Most of all, she is aware that self-care significantly enhances her own work and ability to support others. She also realizes that she is a role model in every respect, including this one.

Finally, Grace possesses the courage and tenacity to investigate and determine what is most true in a given situation. For example, when tapped to be CEO, she was puzzled and serious about her question. Why did they select her?

To find out, she pursued a line of inquiry that most of us miss. Were the skills that helped her in previous roles the same skills that were needed in her new position? She spent several months exploring this question. She found answers by uncovering the complex challenges and opportunities facing the institution. As she learned, she reflected on the knowledge and talents that would be most useful. She sought feedback from trusted others, and she directly asked her new bosses, at appropriate times, how they felt she was doing and what advice they had for her.

During those initial months, she focused on these lessons and began to own the reality of her role. She began to see what she brought to the job and what she needed to let go. The more she accepted the full measure of her fit with the position, the more she relaxed into being herself.

None of us can be a wholly conscious and intentional leader in every waking moment, and Grace is no exception. She is not perfect, yet she is a first-rate example of a leader who deliberately develops, manages, and cares for herself as a leader. Her practices can assist all of us as we develop our own masterful leadership presence.

61

Practice Conscious Influence

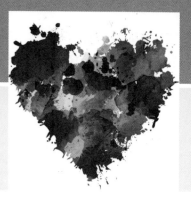

You, the readers of this collection, are the keys to transforming health care and the nursing profession for the future. You do influence future nurse leaders all the time, whether you choose to or not. How can you be more mindful about how you show up, do your work, and impact these leaders-to-be? Every reader is a powerful role model, so here are some tips for assuring that your influence is positive.

At a recent annual meeting of the American Organization for Nursing Leadership, an attendee asked me an important question: "How can nurse leaders make a difference in transforming the nursing profession to meet the needs of the future?" As I consider this question, I am struck by the intense focus that educators, policymakers, and many other national nursing leaders have on the future and how to meet its demands.

I am also aware that every reader of this collection operates in a unique sphere of influence, and within that sphere, every reader has the potential to make a positive—or negative—impact on the future of nursing. That's every reader! So let's tackle the question from that perspective: how can each one of us make a constructive contribution to transforming the future of nursing?

Every nurse leader has one capability that is firmly within his or her grasp. This is one of the highest leverage abilities any leader can employ. It is easy to access, it is always within our control, yet, ironically, many of us fail to use it consistently. This capacity is our *conscious choice*, defined here as our underlying and fundamental ability to *mindfully decide* and then *follow through* on how we are going to show up—that is, how we are going to approach situations, other people, and ourselves at every turn of our lives.

What's the link between this fundamental ability and transforming the nursing profession? The link is that every day, every one of you shape the futures of the newer nurses who cross your path. Your impact may be small or very significant; it may be good or not so good. One thing is certain—you do make an impression. This fact brings with it a choice: you can choose to be a positive influence, or you can be less vigilant. Whichever mode you select, you *will* influence those who are the future of the nursing profession.

Cheryl offers a clear example of just how much a future nursing leader can be shaped by someone who is already a leader. In a recent dialogue, I learned how Cheryl was affected by her "accidental" role model, Maggie, many years ago. When Cheryl first met Maggie, Maggie was an experienced nurse and fellow team member working with Cheryl, a brand new nurse.

Just a few weeks after Cheryl took her first nursing position, one of the patients on her unit had a strong adverse reaction to a medication. The nurses reacted quickly, assembled the medical team, and stabilized the patient. After all the right steps had been taken and the immediate crisis passed, to Cheryl's surprise, Maggie pulled her aside. She asked how Cheryl was feeling about what had just occurred. Cheryl was so impressed with Maggie's concern and their follow-up conversation that she began to politely study Maggie. She observed what Maggie was doing, what she was saying, how she was relating to other people, how she approached patients and tasks, and how she cared for herself. As she viewed Maggie, Cheryl continued to be impressed by Maggie's actions and the values she consistently demonstrated.

This seemingly small exchange led to an experience that profoundly influenced Cheryl. Her story about Maggie helps us understand why today, 10 years later, Cheryl brings the best of her values and professional training to her work without fail. Cheryl is devoted to grooming newer nurses, and she is clear that even when other priorities compete, doing the right thing for patients is her number one concern.

INSPIRING FUTURE NURSE LEADERS

Maggie's actions had a huge impact on a new nurse. Maggie's choices and the actions of many other nurse leaders like her suggest several guidelines for those of us who want to provide positive inspiration for future nurse leaders. We can consciously choose whether we will:

- *Be congruent with our actions, words, and beliefs.* When we act in ways that are not consistent with what we say we value, others notice. Whether we intend to or not, being inconsistent sends the message that we do not mean what we say.
- *Focus on the well-being of those around us, particularly those who are newer to the profession.* Initially, Maggie joined the team that attended to the patient in crisis. Once the crisis had passed, Maggie went to Cheryl and asked how she was doing. That small act let Cheryl know that Maggie cared about how Cheryl was feeling after her first adverse event with a patient. It is important to notice that Maggie was doing anything but "eating her young"!
- *Give generously when we are able.* We don't know what competing commitments Maggie had after this patient event occurred, but we can be sure that there were other demands on her time. Still, she decided to focus on Cheryl first. This choice was generous; Maggie gave of her time and herself.
- *Ask thoughtful questions first.* Maggie approached Cheryl with a question: How was she feeling? Maggie did not start by telling Cheryl about her own feelings. In fact, she did not start by "telling" Cheryl anything at all. She began their dialogue by asking Cheryl about Cheryl. This small gesture sent a big message: Maggie was more interested in hearing about Cheryl's feelings than communicating her own experience first.
- *Explore, don't judge, another person's reactions to a situation.* Maggie's question allowed Cheryl to talk about her experience. As Maggie listened to Cheryl relay her feelings, Cheryl had a very positive reaction. This suggests that Maggie listened with empathy. Maggie's approach to Cheryl is in marked contrast to those who approach us in ways that tell us they are judging us negatively.
- *Monitor our language, words, and tone.* Maggie did not begin her exchange with Cheryl by saying something like, "Wow, that was really terrible, and I've seen it happen far too often up here." Had she opened the dialogue in that way, Maggie would have been venting, unconsciously focusing on herself, and inviting Cheryl to join in her own disaffection with the unit and all its problems. Notice that Maggie still would have influenced Cheryl, but the message and affect would have been entirely different.

As leaders, we can be mindful of those around us who are watching and learning from us all the time—whether we are aware of it or not. We can choose how we show up, and we can realize that we do have an impact. What kind of impact do we want that to be?

62

Know Your Leadership Wake

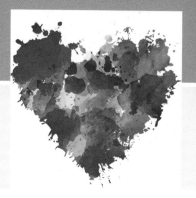

Like it or not, all leaders are influential. The most powerful and effective are those who understand that they have a leadership "wake." A "wake" is the effect, positive and negative, that a leader has on those around her. This column focuses on four thriving nurse leaders who are intentional stewards of their own wakes. We review the qualities these leaders possess and how they manage their influence with aplomb.

In the past year, I have had the honor of serving as the executive coach for four extraordinary nurse leaders. They are from various organizations and locales, and taken together, they offer us great lessons in being conscious stewards of our own power. Their best practices can inform our own, regardless of our rank or position in a health care organization.

These exemplary leaders are aware of their influence and gravitas, or what I call their "leadership wake." A leader's wake is the effect that a leader has on people, and it includes both the positive and negative aspects of their impact. A leader's wake is more than the consequences of his actions; it is also the result of his presence, what he stands for, and what he represents to others.

These leaders are not only mindful of their wakes but also manage them. They know they have a significant influence on the people around them, and they consider how they want to leverage that power. This chapter is about what they do to comport themselves so they create wakes that are, to every extent possible, of their choosing.

Before we review their best practices, let's see how similar and different they are from you and me. Here's a brief overview of their collective leadership profile:

- They are students of their own leadership prowess. This means they are thoughtful witnesses of what goes on around them when they are present. They watch and consider their impact, whether they like this facet of their organizational "persona" or not. They own their power, whether it is derived from their positions, personalities, or both. This does not mean that they act arrogantly or with hubris. It means that they know they are powerful, and they are attentive to how they manage that fact.

- These leaders consider their own presence. They think about what they look like, including their facial expressions and body language. They think about what they wear, how they sound, and the way they walk into a room. This does not mean they think about this constantly, but it does mean that they are aware that these personal characteristics are at least as important, if not more important, than what they say.

- As students of their wakes, these leaders consider them from all sides. They know their words, actions, and presence can have a strongly positive effect on those around them, and they know it can have an equally negative effect. They notice and learn from the circumstances and the actions that beget positive reactions, and those that produce the opposite. For example, they know that sharing their vision or praising their staff will inspire confidence and raise morale among most or all of those who are present. Conversely, they know that an unexplained absence might raise concerns about their support.

- They are also aware that the impact of their presence can be nuanced. Sometimes their words, or lack of them, can evoke uncertainty, lower morale, arouse suspicion, and erode trust. An example of this is when a leader is clearly displeased with the progress of a project but chooses not to say anything. The leader who is conscious of her wake is aware that her facial expression and body language will say it all, whether she utters the words or not. Because she knows this, she usually chooses to be direct and vocal so her words match the overall message that her body language is communicating.

RESPECT AND MASTER YOUR WAKE

So what does this mean for the rest of us? My contention is that if you manage people, you do in fact have a leadership wake. This is true even if you do not have a high-ranking role in your organization or department. When we lead people in any capacity, we affect them in large and small ways. When we are leaders, we are always being watched, whether we like it or not. So it behooves us to learn from exemplary leaders who are masters of their own leadership wakes. Here are some of their best practices:

1. *They realize that effective leadership involves making a claim.* Each of these leaders knows and claims what he or she stands for, and they let that be known to others without hesitation. They are clear about who they are and the organizational values they hold sacred.

2. *They know what they are doing in their roles.* They know and articulate their stake in the ground. This means that they share where they are going, what they are accomplishing, and who they are taking with them. They are attentive to keeping their teams intact, engaged, and inspired to achieve.

3. *They walk tall.* When they enter a room, others know it. Why? They have presence—a palpable energy that attracts people. They carry themselves as if they belong where they are and as if they have something to contribute.

4. *They know when they want to gently evoke the best in others, and they know when they want to more actively provoke the reactions of others.* When they want to engage the best of their team's thinking, they may ask thoughtful, evocative questions that will generate compelling dialogue and innovative solutions. On the other hand, they may choose to be more provocative when they want their colleagues to shift direction.

5. *They know how much space they want to occupy in a given situation.* They are deliberate about times when their silence will facilitate the work, and they know when their voice is needed.

6. *Although they are intentional about the leadership mantles they hold, they are not so taken with their own power that they abuse it.* They know that to do so is to eventually instill distrust and ultimately lose their colleagues' respect.

These leadership practices invite all of us to be more thoughtful about how we are leading, and to notice and attend to the impact we are having. When we lead and manage other people, whether we like it or not, we are definitely having an impact. Bringing our best to our roles requires us to be conscious and thoughtful stewards of our own leadership wakes.

63

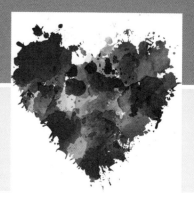

Achieve Success, Again and Again

Thriving nurse leaders don't rest on past accomplishments and old laurels. They don't have to because they know how to repeat their successes. Whether they quell staff discord, revive a faltering team, or turn an organization around, their winning strategy does not end when the incident is over. Masterful leaders and their teams take one final step: they make the time to "harvest" what they learned from what they achieved.

Most of us are familiar with the old adage that we must learn from our mistakes. But how often do we learn from our triumphs? To illustrate this point, this chapter explores two storylines. First, we follow Noel and her team as they achieve an against-all-odds victory. Then we dig underneath to see how they maximized the value of their huge accomplishment. It's the second story that contains valuable lessons for us all.

Let's begin with Noel. When she came into her chief executive officer role 3 years ago, she inherited an organization in turmoil. Its most serious threat was starkly portrayed by outside stakeholders who claimed that the institution no longer had a reason to exist.

Noel also encountered significant problems within her team of senior leaders. They were accomplished individual contributors, but some were in the wrong roles for the work ahead. There were also unhelpful personality clashes that affected the whole team. The group was not a cohesive unit, and it was ill-prepared to lead the organization away from imminent demise.

After gaining a full understanding of her challenges, Noel wasted no time. She partnered with her board and other allies to focus on the organization's mission and determine where it could add value in the new landscape of health care. From there, they developed goals and strategies that held potential for success.

Noel, her board, and the leadership team set about implementing the plan, adjusting as needed during the occasional wins and the many setbacks that followed. Eventually, the number of successes outnumbered the failures, and the organization started to reap the rewards of their intense focus on their updated, mission-consistent contributions. Finally, after nearly 3 years, the organization achieved a new level of viability. Every measure indicated that they had turned the enterprise around.

LEARN FROM YOUR WINS

So, does the story end with "they lived happily ever after"? No. This is where the second story begins. Although it's truly remarkable that Noel and the team achieved a goal that seemed unattainable, the real story is what she and her team did after the organization's trajectory reversed course. *They realized that no matter how great things had become, it wouldn't last. It couldn't. So they were eager to understand and capture what made them successful.* They wanted to embed the learning from their missteps and newfound best practices so they would be ready when future challenges appeared.

What did they discover?

1. *Noel and her team had learned to respect the limits of their professional knowledge.* They now know that it's not enough for leaders to rely on technical, clinical, and health care–specific knowledge. Our organizations and all organizations are in a constant state of change. To survive, we must learn all the time. To make this case, the author Liz Wiseman declares that learning *is* the new knowing.[a] Stated another way, learning trumps knowing, so we must learn how to learn, and we must do it as we go.

2. *Noel and her team realized that they had created a regular practice of cultivating new awareness.* From the start, they had been asking questions about what was working and what wasn't. They did this at the beginning

[a]Wiseman L. *Rookie Smarts: Why Learning Beats Knowing in the New Game of Work.* New York: HarperBusiness; 2014.

when they experienced repeated resistance, and they continued when they had more success. Over time, they developed a culture that was curious rather than judgmental. Instead of saying, "That won't work," they said, "How can we make this work?" If they couldn't find a way, they asked different questions to find new, workable pathways to achieve their goals.

3. **They saw the results of providing resources for team support.** Noel brought in consultants and coaches, they held off-sites, and they invested in knowing who they were individually and as a team.

4. **Noel had support too, and she learned to understand who she was "being" in her role.** The position required her to make difficult calls, particularly regarding the members of the senior team who were in the wrong roles. She also needed to instill a new level of accountability in the team. When she analyzed the skills she needed now, and she compared them with what her previous job required, the two lists were different. In her former role, she had not encountered the destructive power of embedded team dysfunction or her own strong distaste for conflict. Now, Noel had to deal with both. There was simply too much at stake, and she could not default to her old, familiar way of leading.

5. **Noel considered whether she was willing to address the conflicts in the team, implement difficult staffing changes, and build a healthy team.** Of course, she knew the right answers to these questions, but the deeper questions were whether she was equipped for this work and whether she could overcome her aversion to conflict. In the end, she collaborated with her support system and worked to increase her competence in dealing with strife and managing team growth. If we were to query her now about her skill in these areas, she would offer us a realistic assessment—she would say that she is still a "work in progress" on both fronts.

WHAT TYPE OF LEADERSHIP IS NEEDED NOW?

The key lesson for Noel (and for all of us) is to ask what leadership qualities are needed now. Are they what worked in the past, and if not, what do we need to do differently to lead today? If we aren't sure, how can we find out? Once we know, how can we develop those skills? Equally important, what will help us access our capacity for valor and courage so we can lead differently when we don't know, and can't know, all the answers?

The good news is that Noel changed the composition of the team, and over time, its members learned to support one another. This was most evident when the organization offered its premier programs. The team learned to operate interdependently to produce their large, now-successful offerings. This was not easy for these decidedly independent individual contributors. Despite the difficulty, over time, this formerly dysfunctional team gelled. But to get there, they went through several iterations of forming, storming, and norming. Now the team's self-described "new normal" is what they all claim is "performing."[b]

The team learned in the moment by asking questions. They did this before, during, and after signal events. They developed practices to reflect on and talk about themselves and their work as a team and as individuals working together. They acknowledged and celebrated their achievements and learning, and they admitted their setbacks.

Significantly, the laughter on the team increased exponentially as they became more unified. Although they know that their very big organization-wide victory is a treasured moment in time, they are confident about their newfound capacity to learn, grow, and change together. They know they can rely on this critical skill as they weather the storms they have yet to face.

[b]Tuckman B. Developmental sequence in small groups. *Psychol Bull.* 1965:63;384–399.

Epilogue

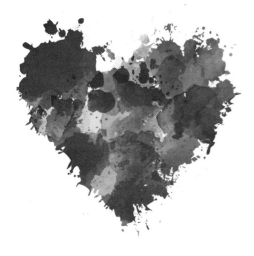

It is my fervent hope that this collection has offered you inspiration as well as a road map for leading with mastery and heart—regardless of your career stage. Here is one final chapter to help you make the most of your "coaching," whether you received it from this collection or from any other coaching source. I include this because many of us experience wonderful leadership learning opportunities, only to rush back into the demands of our daily work lives. When we do this, it is all too easy for fresh learning to be pushed aside and even extinguished. In this last article, "Make the Most of Coaching," I offer ways for you to reflect on and "install" the new insights and practices that your coaching has provided you.

64

Make the Most of Coaching

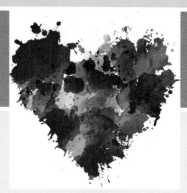

How many times have you been excited about fresh learning and spot-on insights, only to return to the harsh reality of the old problems you left behind? How many times have too much work and a demanding personal life quickly and permanently dulled your innovative ideas and dampened your motivation to use them?

Most of us experience the highs and lows of leadership development, regardless of the venue: conference, seminar, or on-the-job training. But the challenges of sustaining novel approaches to managing and leading can be even bigger when a coaching relationship comes to an end. Whether we've been in team or individual coaching, as "coachees," we may worry that our new knowledge won't stick when the support and discipline of formal coaching end.

Most of us thrive in customized coaching relationships that offer us the chance for personal reflection and solutions that are tailored to our unique needs. When these arrangements conclude, we may think that what we've achieved is because of the coach, even though we are the ones who tried out new behaviors and created better outcomes. Although good coaches can be sage and timely guides, these same good coaches will be the first to say that we are not dependent on them to keep growing as a leader.

One case in point is Rich, the rural health nurse executive who inspired a Coaching Forum chapter entitled "What Do You Choose to Animate?"[a] Rich's leadership life

was fraught with a heavy workload, constant change, a lot of travel, and health and interpersonal challenges. Rich was a capable executive, but the excesses in his work life proved a lot for him to handle, so when he came to coaching, he was eager to transform his thinking and ways of working.

One of his early realizations was that he was focusing on all the wrong things—he was letting his own stories of the insurmountable bigness of his position script the increasingly difficult challenges of his job and much of his life. In his coaching, he learned to notice this and reframe his thinking; he no longer enlivened the worst of his feelings and his own fatalistic renditions of his work environment.

He also learned to let go of his strong wish for perfect solutions to complex and intractable problems.

Rich learned a great deal in his coaching, but when it was time to end the engagement, he feared that he would lose his momentum and his new leadership ways. So, he asked for his final coaching session to focus on how to sustain what he had learned. Here is what Rich's post-coaching "tool box" looked like. As you review it, keep in mind that this list can easily be modified to apply to any significant learning journey.

Make a short, succinct list of the major takeaways from your coaching. Create the list in a language that is meaningful and memorable for you, regardless of whether the coach used these terms or not. Reflect on what you've written and remember the key ideas in the days and weeks to come. You might want to post this brief list on your mirror or at your workstation as a daily reminder.

1. ***Celebrate your success.*** Appreciate your own hard work, discipline, and coaching accomplishments. Give yourself the credit and acknowledgment you deserve.

---

[a]Robinson-Walker, C. Chapter 8 *in Leading with Mastery and Heart: A Coaching Companion for Thriving Nurse Leaders.* St. Louis, MO: Elsevier; 2020.

2. ***As you go forward, prioritize reflection on a daily basis*** if you can, or a weekly basis if you can't do it more frequently. Consider how you are leading now: Are you employing what you learned? Are you adjusting and strengthening it? Or are you reverting to old habits that don't serve you or others? Remember that reflection will be especially important if you are action oriented and/or if your position is highly demanding. In these circumstances, it is all too easy to be swept up in busyness. Then, your old ways will return, and even the best coaching outcomes will fade quickly.

3. ***Remember that slips happen.*** If you find yourself reverting to old reactions and patterns, take comfort in knowing that it's normal. We all do this when learning new leadership skills. We all need to practice and then practice some more. We can't acquire the uniquely polished versions of our new behaviors until we experiment, try them in different circumstances, and occasionally even fail at applying them appropriately. What's important about slips is that they are opportunities for learning and change. We can consider why our effort didn't work, and what we will do differently the next time.

4. ***Remember what was most helpful about your coaching.*** Was it the structure of regular meetings? Was it having the opportunity to speak confidentially with someone knowledgeable? Was it having an accountability partner who was supporting you? How can you bring the most useful aspects of coaching into your post-coaching life?

5. ***Develop a plan for continued learning.*** What would you like to learn in the next quarter? What skill could you improve that will have the greatest impact on your career and leadership? What learning goals would you like to set for yourself and how will you achieve them?

6. ***Engage with a learning partner.*** Be explicit about what you want from the relationship: perhaps it's a listening, nonjudgmental "ear"; perhaps it's someone to respectfully challenge your thinking or behavior; perhaps it's someone to help you stay on track and remind you of your goals.

7. ***Watch your positive role models.*** Let them inspire you.

8. ***Keep practicing.*** Don't relegate your hard-earned leadership growth to the "over and done" category, and put it on the shelf. As we all know too well, fresh learning is short-lived if we don't practice and refine it.

This is a big array of options to keep learning alive when a formal coaching relationship ends. Like any tool box, you won't use all these components all the time, but if you select those that are most helpful, you will be well positioned to benefit from your coaching for many years to come.

Coaching Forum Paying Tribute to Dr. Angeles Arrien

Catherine Robinson-Walker, MBA, MCC
The Coaching Forum April 2014

1541-4612/2014, Copyright 2014 by Elsevier Inc., All rights reserved. https://dx.doi.org/10.1016/j.mnl.2014.07.008

While it is always a pleasure to write this column for the *Nurse Leader*, this time the occasion is both joyous and sad. In this issue, I am honoring the life of Angeles Arrien, PhD, who passed away in April 2014. Angeles was a cultural anthropologist and a true "shaman" whose work and wisdom graced many nurse leaders, including those in the Center for Nursing Leadership (CNL), sponsored by Hill-Rom, AONE (Formerly the American Organization of Nurse Executives), and the Network for Healthcare Management from 1995 through the early 2000s.

Angeles was best known for her authorship of *The Four-Fold Way: Walking the Paths of the Warrior, Teacher, Healer, and Visionary.*[1] This book, filled with heart and deep wisdom, was just one of her many contributions to any field, and most particularly the field of leadership. In this and other works, Angeles revealed her unique capacity to understand the principles of native people from many traditions. She was able to translate them into insights that are relevant in any modern setting that requires exceptional stewardship.

Although it is impossible to capture the full spectrum of Angeles' knowledge in this short piece, I would like to offer a few highlights. In addition to reading her works in the CNL, I had the privilege of working directly with Angeles as my personal coach from 2005 through 2007. Here are some of the insights I gained from those experiences.

1. Angeles encouraged us, as leaders, to focus on what we want to see in the world, not what is wrong with what we see in the world.
2. Long before it became fashionable, Angeles foresaw a world of mutuality and collaboration versus a world in which one leader or one tribe or one culture is deemed "better than" or "superior to" another.
3. Angeles offered strategies for managing conflict that were profound in their simplicity:
   a. Show up
   b. Follow what has heart and meaning
   c. Tell the truth without blame or judgment
   d. Be open to outcome versus attached to outcome
4. She talked about the "shadow archetype" of a visionary, which is self-abandonment. She also suggested why some leaders embody this negative way of being:
   a. For others' love
   b. For others' acceptance and approval
   c. To maintain balance
   d. To stay in a state of harmony
5. Angeles pointed out that nature's rhythm is medium slow. As mammals born of nature, we are not built for a world that is perpetually fast paced and focused on multitasking. It is up to us to slow down and to listen to and honor what our bodies tell us. At times, it is up to us to be patient and wait for what is emerging, even when what is emerging is not yet clear.
6. As leaders, when we are dependent on action, and only action, we are denying the wisdom that comes from slowing down to understand who we are "being" in a given situation.

Those familiar with Angeles knew of her profound commitment to authenticity and to the importance of living a life that reflects our essential spirits. To that end, she counseled us to notice:

- What genuinely inspires us, and to follow those sources wherever they lead.
- What energizes us versus what depletes us. When we are open to these insights, we are engaged with our own truth, and we can act from a place of belief in ourselves and the world around us.

- The difference between overachieving and perfectionism versus excellence. She understood that the overachiever does not trust her own gifts. The leader striving for perfection is coming from a basis of fear. By contrast, excellence is about showing up with a full heart, doing our best, and coming from a position of trust. Choosing excellence allows us to relax and to lead with commitment and courage.

Angeles said that learning to trust life is one of the most central lessons any of us can learn. This belief has some deeply important elements:

1. There are significant differences between attempting to control and allowing ourselves to trust. The same is true for struggling versus trusting. Recognizing these distinctions is important for any leader. They are important to us personally as well, especially as we enter the second half of life.
2. She asked that we examine the relationship we have with our own "voice"—our own wisdom. Do we trust it? Or do we have a "conditional relationship" with our own truth?

Throughout Angeles Arrien's life, she was unflinchingly committed to integrity. This deeply resonated with me because of my own research on the significance of integrity in perceived leadership effectiveness for health care leaders.[2] As Angeles noted in *The Four-Fold Way,* "many societies recognize that a lack of alignment between word and action results in a loss of power and effectiveness."[2(p.16)] Angeles was passionate about being consistent in thought and deed. She believed that by nurturing our own congruence and wholeness we can live in integrity and fully attend to our leadership and the real meaning of our own life story. I am deeply grateful for Dr. Angeles Arrien and the gifts she gave to all of us.

REFERENCES

1. Arrien, A. (1993). *The four-fold way: Walking the paths of the warrior, teacher, healer, and visionary.* San Francisco: Harper San Francisco.
2. Robinson-Walker, C. (1999). *Women and leadership in healthcare: The journey to authenticity and power.* San Francisco: Jossey-Bass.

INDEX